# The Mindful Parent

# The Mindful Parent

STRATEGIES FROM PEACEFUL
CULTURES TO RAISE COMPASSIONATE,
COMPETENT KIDS

Charlotte Peterson, PhD

Skyhorse Publishing

Skyhorse Publishing books may be purchased in bulk at special discounts for sales promotion, corporate gifts, fund-raising, or educational purposes. Special editions can also be created to specifications. For details, contact the Special Sales Department, Skyhorse Publishing, 307 West 36th Street, 11th Floor, New York, NY 10018 or info@skyhorsepublishing.com.

Skyhorse® and Skyhorse Publishing® are registered trademarks of Skyhorse Publishing, Inc.®, a Delaware corporation.

Visit our website at www.skyhorsepublishing.com.

10 9 8 7 6 5 4 3 2 1

Library of Congress Cataloging-in-Publication Data is available on file.

ISBN: 978-1-63450-446-1

Ebook ISBN: 978-1-6345-0464-5

Printed in the United States of America

**To Dr. Vivian Olum:**
Who taught me about listening to a child.

**To Grandma Dina:**
Who taught me about being cherished as a child.

**To Julie Gerald:**
Who taught me about loving a child.

**To Shane and Emily:**
Who continue teaching me about being a better mother . . .

**To Ellis and Oliver:**
Who are just arriving to escort me into
the whole new world of being a Grammy . . .

**And:**
To all the parents in the world who showed me how to nurture children.
To them I owe great gratitude, as I would have been a much less
kind and patient parent without their examples.

*People often ask me what is the most effective technique*
*For transforming their lives.*
*It is a little embarrassing after years and years of*
*Research and experimentation,*
*I have to say that the best answer is—*
*Just be a little kinder.*
—Aldous Huxley


*Three things in human life are important...*
*The first is to be kind.*
*The second is to be kind.*
*The third is to be kind.*
—Mother Teresa

# Table of Contents

# Table of Contents

# Introduction

*It's not our job to toughen our children up to face a cruel and heartless world.*
*It's our job to raise children who will make the world a little less cruel and heartless.*
—L. R. Knost

Have you ever wondered how kind people got that way? Anyone who has gazed into a newly born baby's eyes knows that the very essence of human nature is a deeply profound yearning to form a close, loving relationship. Kindness is not something that needs to be taught; it's something that needs to be protected and nurtured from the beginning of life. Parenting practices in peaceful cultures have much to teach us about preserving this precious desire for connection that resides inside every newborn. When parents open their hearts and respond sensitively to their infants, kind, joyful, and trusting children are the result.

Children in this country, however, are not faring so well. Currently, twenty percent of all kids in the United States are being diagnosed with a psychological disorder. The United States uses *ninety percent* of all the medications in the world that are given to children for mental health issues. The suicide rate of children has doubled in the past twenty years. There is also a dramatic increase in the severity of bullying. We even have kids using firearms to kill parents, teachers, and other children. This current epidemic of childhood psychological distress, aggression, and bullying has got to be understood so it can be reversed. (See the Appendix for "Indicators of Children in Crisis.")

Parenting practices are usually culturally-based: learned from our parents (for better or worse), pediatricians (who are typically not trained in children's emotional needs), and the popular "how-to" parenting books of the day. As a psychologist for the past thirty-five years, I have found that the majority of my clients carry painful early memories concerning how they were parented, although I have never encountered parents who intentionally wanted to harm their children. A serious disconnect seems to exist between accepted parenting practices and actual understanding of children's needs. The way babies are treated from the very beginning leaves an imprint on their self-esteem, overall happiness, and comfort with relationships throughout their lives. While most parents deeply love their children, many have trouble showing their youngsters, even when babies, the most important ingredient: that they are completely and unconditionally cherished. (Reference to *babies* includes the time during pregnancy, birth, and the first three years of life.)

In my early twenties, I began traveling and immersing myself in other cultures. Initially, I was just excited to be exploring the world, but I soon began to focus on the children I encountered along the way and how they were being parented. It is usually believed that the way something is done in one's country of origin is the way it should be done, and I had never considered there were other ways to raise children. I was, in fact, astonished to witness how differently youngsters were being parented in some parts of the world. Especially noticeable was the closeness mothers seemed to have with their infants and toddlers. Not only were babies being breastfed, something that was quite foreign to my American eyes in the 1970s, but also they were constantly worn on their mother's bodies, responded to quickly, and seemed delightfully calm and content. In many Western countries, it has traditionally been frowned upon to quickly tend to crying babies, due to the fear that infants would become "spoiled" if given too much attention. I had assumed that babies everywhere were treated similarly by their busy parents and spent much time alone often fussing in cribs, playpens, and highchairs. I quickly realized this was not the case, and began questioning if there is actually a "right" or "best" way to parent infants and toddlers. Since all human babies are biologically the same, could different parenting styles produce children who were more joyful, gentle, and caring?

This question began my lifelong pursuit of observing babies throughout the world, attempting to understand which parenting practices create the most positive relationships and the most enjoyable, kind children. I have spent three to six months every five years for the past four decades living in a different part of the world and, to date, have observed parenting in over sixty countries and on nearly every continent. During the past twenty-five years, I have focused my travels on cultures that have a history of being nonviolent. Spending time with Tibetan, Balinese, and Bhutanese parents, I am convinced that their close parent-child relationships beginning from preconception, along with their extremely gentle, attentive, and compassionate nurturing of newborns and toddlers, do indeed grow kinder kids.

*The Mindful Parent* shares parenting wisdom I have gathered from indigenous parents, grandparents, professionals, and village leaders that help infants and toddlers become more self-reliant, cooperative, happy, and caring children. Extensive interviews providing excerpts, which are scattered throughout this book, were conducted in Bhutan, Bali, Japan, and the Tibetan community in Northern India. To the people of nonviolent cultures I owe great gratitude. Numerous parents, including myself, have raised delightfully kind children following their examples.

Mindful Parenting is a blend of parenting practices that I have developed over four decades of studying child development, helping clients heal from childhood traumas, observing parents throughout the world, and experimenting with these techniques as a mother with my own son and daughter. Mindful Parenting involves being aware, engaged, and responsive to your children's needs, with the ultimate goal of creating close, mutually-compassionate relationships. Mindful Parenting of Infants details globally observed parenting practices that lead to wonderfully loving attachments between parents and their infants. Mindful Parenting of Toddlers involves helping babies from about eighteen months of age become mindful of their ability to control their own behavior through a unique process of introspective discipline called Time-In. Cultures that practice Mindful Parenting have children with a high degree of self-control, self-esteem, cooperation, generosity, and empathy.

Attachment is the most important key to parenting your children. Feeling closely attached to your infant means not just loving her, but also feeling "in love" with her. We all know that when we are "in love" with someone, we are willing to give them as much help as we possibly can when they are distressed. While it is impossible to meet every one of your baby's needs and there is no such thing as a perfect parent, your attitude is what matters most. Understanding that human infants are born completely helpless, not able to even scratch their own itches, and they cry to desperately summon help, will make it easier to respond more positively than if you believe their cries are meant to manipulate you or thoughtlessly ruin your night's sleep. Closely attached parents do their best to understand what is wrong and then respond in sensitive, caring ways. Rest assured that if you parent in this way, your infant will know you care even at those times when you can't respond immediately or have no idea why she is upset. The short pause between her crying out for help and your response will usually not escalate into loud screaming when she learns to anticipate that you will be there soon to help her. Saying, "I can't come right now, but will be there as soon as I can," or "I don't know what's wrong, but I'm right here with you," communicates a far different message than, "You're such a demanding kid. I'm not letting your cries control me!"

Some parents wonder whether it is best to raise children who are tough, competitive, and self-focused, believing that those qualities will make their children more resilient to life's challenges. The opposite has actually been found to be true. Scientific research confirms that kind people are healthier, happier, and have greater success in their relationships and careers.[1] Kindness does not simply mean always being nice, it means caring about how your actions affect others. Kind people seem better able to deal with and heal from life stresses because they tend to have more social support and can communicate their feelings and needs rather than becoming helplessly isolated. Current research on early brain development in babies confirms that extensive nurturing during infancy is critical for optimal brain development and increases the child's ability to be self-calming, kind, and emotionally resilient.

Paid parental leave with guaranteed job protection is available in almost all countries throughout the world after the birth or adoption of a baby. In many developed countries, paid leave is provided to parents for one to three years. This kind of support greatly improves the opportunity for parents to have close attachments with their babies, including extensive nurturing and extended breastfeeding. While such governmental support is not available in the United States, yet (we must remain hopeful), the final chapter of this book offers parents unique ideas to help them find a balance between their financial, career, and young children's needs.

Introduction

Inspiring interviews are provided by parents and grandparents who were willing to share intimate details about their parenting stresses and the major lifestyle changes they are making to ensure their infants and toddlers are getting the early emotional support they need.

Just trying to understand your infant's needs will help him feel worthy of being loved. And by continually listening to your baby, he ultimately will teach you what he needs and how best to be his parent. Creating a close connection with your infant will make the toddler years, when you need to set limits, encourage patience, and teach appropriate behavior, go much more smoothly. The overall most important goal for parenting is to build and protect your relationship with your kids and try to reconnect with them whenever you feel disconnected. Such mindful parenting will not only be more enjoyable, but will result in growing kind kids, happy families, positive schools, safe communities, more nonviolent societies, and hopefully, a more peaceful world.

*If we hope to create a nonviolent world*
*Where respect and kindness replace fear and hatred,*
*We must begin with how we treat each other*
*at the beginning of life,*
*For that is where our deepest patterns are set.*
*From these roots grow fear and alienation*
*or love and trust.*
—Suzanne Arms

# CHAPTER 1

# Parenting Lessons
# From Around the World

*There can be no keener revelation of a society's soul
than the way in which it treats its children.*

—Nelson Mandela

After spending my childhood dreaming of seeing the world, in 1974 I strapped a backpack on my twenty-eight-year-old shoulders and set off on a fourteen-month honeymoon adventure with my husband, Carl. Our goal was to travel and live among the people of Mexico, Central America, and South America. I especially wanted to experience the indigenous Aztecan, Mayan, and Incan cultures.

Immediately obvious was that the children "south of the border" were being parented very differently than they were back home in the US. Infants were worn in front slings on their mother's body, breastfed whenever they whimpered, and continuously kept in close contact throughout the day. Toddlers were carried on their mother's back, where they could be easily comforted by soft, soothing voices. Youngsters continued to be breastfed and took naps on their mothers' bodies until they were at least four years old. These children were calm, content, and clearly thriving. I suddenly began to question what I learned about raising children from my family and most of my psychology classes. Recalling the words of Erik Erikson, an early developmental psychologist, I wondered if this was the type of parenting to which he was referring. Erikson had been adamant that for a child to develop a "sense of trust" in relationships, it required "sensitive care of the baby's individual needs."[1]

My major lifetime quest became to observe parenting practices throughout the world. In order to accomplish this goal we arranged our lives so that every five years, our family would travel to a different

1

part of the world and live there for three to six months. Over a period of forty years, we lived throughout the Americas, Europe, Near East, South Pacific, Africa, and Central and Southeast Asia.

In India, Thailand, Nepal, and Tanzania I observed similar mother-infant relationships to what I had seen earlier in Central and South America. Even in the world's poorest countries, mothers were continually doing their best to meet the emotional needs of their babies. Infants and toddlers were worn on their mother's body, breastfed at will, kept in close contact during the day, and bed-shared with their parents at night. While no culture is perfect or has all the best answers for raising children, observing parents and children in other countries exposed me to new possibilities that opened my mind to wondering which parenting practices truly help babies thrive. Basic biological needs of babies are the same everywhere in the world; it is the local customs of infant and toddler care that vary greatly. So, which ones promote optimum development and support infants in reaching their greatest physical, mental, and emotional potentials?

## Parenting in Truly Peaceful Cultures

Fifteen years after traveling throughout much of the world, I decided to focus on visiting cultures that had made political and spiritual commitments to nonviolence. The peaceful cultures in which I've enjoyed observing parenting are the Tibetan, Bhutanese, and Balinese. My quest has been to discover how children are cared for in these cultures and whether there seems to be a connection between parenting practices and growing people who are more peace loving and compassionate. Simply put, I wondered if the way babies are treated in these cultures contributes to growing kinder kids. What I have seen makes me believe that this is indeed the case. In these peaceful cultures, there is great attentiveness, extended nurturing, and more rituals honoring infants and young children than I have observed anywhere else in the world. The children appear much calmer, confident, joyful, and kind (see photo 1).

Another consistent difference in these cultures seems to be more social equality and respect between men and women with recognition of how genders differ and can complement each other. This appreciation of differences, rather than competition between the genders, results in mothers and fathers more comfortably sharing the caregiving of their children. Throughout history, there is evidence that nonviolent cultures have been more gender-balanced with equal respect for males and females, such as the Semai people of Malaysia,[2] and the ancient Minoan society on the island of Crete, where people are believed to have lived peacefully for fifteen hundred years.[3]

## Tibetan

In 1959, at the young age of twenty-four, the leader of the Tibetan people, His Holiness the Dalai Lama, was put to the critical test of whether he would truly follow his spiritual commitment to nonviolence. As the Chinese invasion into Tibet was occurring, the Dalai Lama chose fleeing in exile to India over resorting to fighting a war. He maintained that if the Tibetans killed others in order to keep their homeland, they could no longer live there with open hearts, peace of mind, and compassion for all beings, beliefs that are the foundation of their Buddhist spiritual teachings.[4] The Dalai Lama was given protection in northern India where he has lived since that time, having been joined by more than one hundred thousand Tibetans who also have fled their homeland to follow him. For the past fifty-five years, the "Tibetan Government in Exile" has been sharing its nonviolent teachings with people throughout the world.

The Tibetans continue to strive for gender equality, honoring the importance of mothering, along with fathers having specific roles in helping to nurture their children. The Tibetans have great reverence for mothering. They consider mother-love during the early months and years of a child's life to be the primary source for the development of compassion. The Dalai Lama believes that females are naturally more emotionally sensitive and a mother's emotional state directly influences her child's mind during the pregnancy, continues throughout breastfeeding, and on into the relationship that grows between them.[5] The Dalai Lama is certain that we learn how to love from our mothers, and this first relationship sets the tone for all future relationships (see photo 2). "You cannot compare the mother's care with anyone else's care. In other words, mother's care and love for you is the epitome of love."[6] The Dalai Lama, winner of the 1989 Nobel Peace Prize, is considered to be one of the most compassionate people alive today. When asked how he became such a kind person, he warmly acknowledges that he learned compassion, caring, and devotion from his mother. The Dalai Lama's youngest brother has said, "The tremendous warmth that I feel toward my mother and the warmth she gave me, I think, is the greatest gift I ever received."[7]

The Tibetans refer to an ancient book, with information said to be three thousand years old that details every week of pregnancy. It offers advice as to what expectant parents can do to optimize the physical and emotional development of their fetus. The importance of these ancient Tibetan beliefs are now being validated by early brain research in developed countries.[8]

Tibetans have seven stages of early child rearing: *Preconception, Conception, Gestation, Birthing, Bonding, Infancy,* and *Early Childhood.* Extensive rituals and specific parenting practices are conducted during each of these stages.[9] It is notable that five of these stages occur before infancy, the point at which most Westerners tend to think parenting begins.

The importance of preparing for conception, something that the Tibetans have long known, is just beginning to be realized in the US. After a young Tibetan couple marries and before they become pregnant, groundwork begins to help create an infant who will be healthy in mind and body. *Preconception* is a time to prepare the body, mind, and emotions to welcome the spirit of a child. The young couple is instructed to cleanse their bodies of any toxins, to eat healthy food, and to cleanse their minds of any negativities, such as anger, greed, hatred, and jealousy. For centuries, Tibetans have known that negative emotions in the mother can alter the brain development of the gestating baby. Western neuroscientists are confirming that a mother who feels relatively calm and secure during pregnancy helps to create a baby with a larger forebrain (higher reasoning and social awareness) rather than an enlarged hindbrain (basic survival and flight-fight response).[10]

Tibetans consider *Conception* a sacred event for which a couple should prepare and plan. The couple is encouraged to consciously invite a baby to enter during a gentle and loving union.

During the period of *Gestation*, the father has an especially significant role. He is expected to give his wife and unborn baby as much love and care as possible in order to increase positive feelings in the pregnant mother, thereby positively affecting the biochemistry within the developing fetus. *The Tibetan Art of Parenting* (1997) explains that "Each week of gestation holds evolutionary developments, which, when attended to, can guide parents to make choices that assist, rather than hinder, the life unfolding in the womb."[11]

All friends and members of the extended family are involved in some way during the *Birthing* stage, which is usually a natural homebirth with a midwife. Everyone comforts and nurtures the birthing woman while eagerly awaiting the opportunity to welcome the cherished newborn. Each step in the process (labor, delivery, birth, and postpartum) is celebrated with specific rituals and ancient traditions.

Immediately after the birth, the baby is kept with the mother and this period is regarded as a sacred time of *Bonding* between the parents and infant. Following the birth it is considered important for immediate family members to spend the first few days only with each other. Fathers are very involved with household chores and care of the family so the new mother can rest and closely attach to her newborn.[12] Tibetans believe that during this bonding period, the most powerful way that the baby feels his mother's love is through breastfeeding. So, it is important that the mother cultivate positive feelings of love toward her suckling infant. If the mother has feelings of resentment, it is believed that they also will get fed directly to the nursing baby. Nursing mothers refrain from the use of alcohol, nicotine, and caffeine, just as they did during preconception and pregnancy; it is understood "that these substances, passed to their babies through their milk, could damage their children's bodies and minds."[13]

Babies are believed to have abilities, sensitivities, and heightened perceptions during their *Infancy* stage that adults no longer possess. Mothers are rarely separated from their babies, who are always in arms or worn on the front or back of their mother's body. Tibetans consider touch and continuous bodily contact to be especially important for bonding and brain development, so someone is always holding and caressing the baby.

The *Early Childhood* stage is considered a very special time for nurturing in Tibetan children's lives. Infants and toddlers are always responded to when they cry. Children spend their days with a loved family member, are breastfed for many years, and sleep with their parents until about seven years of age. Ritualized celebrations at each developmental milestone in a child's early life are believed to encourage positive physical, mental, emotional, and spiritual growth. Parents teach their children through modeling, memorization, and movement to help the information be integrated both intellectually and intuitively.[14] Educating the heart along with the mind is highly valued for both boys and girls. A Tibetan explained to me that the more educated boys are, the better husbands and fathers they later become. The Dalai Lama states, "Although from an ideal perspective human qualities ought to be developed in conjunction with kindness, I often say that if I had to choose between important general qualities and kindness, I believe I would choose kindness."[15]

When I ask people from Western countries what their goal is for parenting, common responses are that they want to raise a child who is independent, productive, successful, happy, and wealthy. When the same question is asked of Tibetans, the answer given is to raise a child who is as wise, generous, and compassionate as possible. Tibetan boys and girls are encouraged to be non-aggressive and empathetic to all living beings (including even the smallest insects). Just imagine how greatly parenting practices might differ depending on one's goals for their children.

During a December 1994 trip to India, I had the great fortune of spending an entire evening with Rinchen Khando Choegyal, sister-in-law of the Dalai Lama, and the minister of education for the Tibetan Government in Exile, as well as the first president of the Tibetan Woman's Association. The two of us sat huddled by a makeshift woodstove in the home built for the Dalai Lama's mother, trying to warm ourselves against the Himalayan winter chill. We talked of our own children and of mothering in our two cultures.

Rinchen Khando has been given the task of creating more educational and career-oriented opportunities for Tibetan women, in-line with the Dalai Lama's commitment to establishing even greater equality between the genders. She asked me if I had any suggestions of how this could be done without the children getting hurt from not enough mothering.[16] She stressed that the importance of mother-love in creating a trusting, kind child must not be underestimated. It is understood by Tibetans that when a woman chooses to become a mother, "bringing a precious new human being into this world is the most wonderful and challenging responsibility of her entire life."[17]

After carefully considering her question, I answered that great changes had been made in the US during the 1970s with respect to women's rights and career opportunities. I stated, however, that we were unaware of the importance that nurturing played in infant development and believed that at a few months of age babies could be cared for just as well in day care centers. Because of this, I added, many children had probably not gotten adequate attention from their mothers.

Rinchen Khando respectfully acknowledged that she suspected American babies had been hurt by this lack of time with their mothers and pondered if perhaps it could be the reason so many problems exist between parents and teenagers in the US. She expressed sorrow about this occurrence, adding that possibly other cultures could learn from this and make adjustments so that young children would receive the nurturing they truly need.[18]

That was the crystallizing moment when this book was conceived. This gentle, sincere woman in a remote Indian village seemed more aware of familial problems in our culture than most of us in the US. I realized it was imperative to share the information about parenting practices that I had observed throughout the world, especially concerning the importance of nurturing infants and toddlers.

## Bhutanese

The Kingdom of Bhutan is a landlocked country high in the Himalayan Mountains that has had a long history of nonviolence. This peaceful culture has been protected from Western influence by five genera-tions of highly educated, benevolent, environmentally conscious kings chosen because they have been especially gifted at compromise and negotiation. In 1972, Bhutan's former King Jigme Singye Wangchuck introduced the concept of "Gross National Happiness" (GNH) in an attempt to define what qualities of life promote human happiness, as differentiated from "Gross Domestic Product" (GDP), which is solely based on economic prosperity.[19]

Getting into Bhutan is not easy; very few visas are given to Western-ers traveling without an organized tour group. During a trip to India in 2004, I persevered through numerous visa denials before finally receiving permission to visit Bhutan for five days. What an honor and delight to spend time in this country! When government officials understood that gathering information about parenting was the purpose of my trip, I was kindly introduced to parents, doctors, and educators. Bhutan is an egali-tarian culture in which there is much equality between men and women. Women are not only equally educated to men and hold jobs of respect, but as a matrilineal culture, the mother is considered the head of the fam-ily, and all familial inheritances pass to the women of the family.[20]

Pediatrician Mimi Lhamu explained to me, while nursing her own infant son, that babies in Bhutan are given lots of loving care and treated with great respect. Infants are always breastfed for at least two years. When a woman chooses to return to her job (sometimes when the infant is only three months old), usually the maternal grandmother cares for the baby during the day and takes the baby to its mother twice a day to be nursed. If the new mother's own mother is not able to care for the child, then an older woman with the specific qualification being one "who truly loves babies" is chosen to care for the infant in their home.[21]

Fathers and older siblings are also very involved in caring for the babies. I often saw older brothers carrying and playing with their young-est siblings. Babies are always responded to when they cry, and no one would ever consider hitting a child.

Infants and toddlers accompany their parents to work whenever pos-sible (see photo 3). In the local shoe shop, I observed a three-year-old boy taking a nap on one of the shelves behind his father's checkout stand.

In the US, if we have a similar job, why wouldn't we consider taking our babies or toddlers to work?

## Balinese

A culture whose long-held commitment to nonviolence has recently been put to a stringent test is the Balinese. In October 2002, there was a terrible terrorist attack on Bali in which a popular nightclub was bombed. Over two hundred young tourists and local Balinese people died, and hundreds more suffered horrific injuries. A fire spread for miles burning everything in its wake. I was told that young Balinese males at the scene of the attack wanted to find who had done this and kill them. A Balinese elder sternly stopped the young men. He is reported to have divided the boys into three subgroups telling one third of them to go to the bombsite and pick up body parts. He sent the second group to the hospital to help the burn victims. The third group was told to go to the morgue to help people identify their loved ones. Then the elder told the young men to return to him the following evening and let him know if they wanted to cause this kind of pain to someone else.[22]

Elder wisdom of this type is what young people need in order to see beyond the immediate desire for revenge. That wise elder was able to stop a cycle of violence by transforming feelings of aggression into those of responsibility, caregiving, and compassion. The Balinese hold fast to these values. But, how do they become people who are able to make such incredible moral leaps? During my five visits over the past twenty-five years, I have spent nearly twelve months living in Bali. I truly believe that the emotional foundation for becoming such peaceful people is shaped by how the Balinese are treated from the beginning of their lives.

The Balinese have a spiritual practice that does not exist elsewhere. It is a hybrid of Hinduism, Buddhism, and the Animistic religion of the indigenous people of Bali. Their belief that an infant is a spiritual gift from the heavens, who is most likely a reincarnation of a previously loved family member, sets the foundation for the close parent-infant relationship. Imagine how it would feel to be born into a culture where babies are cherished and thought of as "pure goodness" and "close to the gods." Where you were respected as the most honored member of the family. Where you would be constantly held in someone's arms for the first three months of your life, with everyone longing to hold and care for you just to soak up some of your heavenly energy. If reincarnation does exist, this is where I would wish to be reborn.

Bali is truly my "heart-home." I have observed an entire generation in "my village" mature over two and a half decades—adults have become elders, teens are now the village leaders, and children have become parents with babies of their own. Learning the basics of the Bahasa Indonesian language made it easier to do my research and allowed me to have close relationships with a Balinese family who has "adopted" me as a family member. To this day, I am treated with respect and love, while being addressed with the most honored title: "*Ibu*," meaning, "mother."

Many things have changed in Bali since my first trip there in 1989. The village now has electricity, people ride motorbikes instead of bicycles, most adults have cell phones, and there are fewer rice fields due to land being used for cafés and tourist bungalows. While the economy suffered greatly after the terrorist bombing made tourists reluctant to visit, the people of Bali have continued to have the happiest smiles and kindest hearts of any people I have met on this planet (see photo 4).

When living among the Balinese, one quickly realizes that these people are unusually joyful and kindhearted. Their degree of compassion is striking. I once asked an older man why Balinese people were so generous. His confusing response was that people are generous because they are very selfish. He went on to explain that if he did something to make me happy, it made him feel good inside; but if he did something that hurt me, he wouldn't be able to sleep at night. So, he delightfully concluded that by making me happy he was doing the same for himself, and smilingly added that he was therefore actually being selfish. Abiding by this simple, but profound understanding of empathy makes for positive relationships. A few days into our first trip to Bali, my daughter, Emily, who was five years old, asked, "How did these people *get* so happy?" She followed this a few days later with, "Don't babies here know how to cry?"

Balinese rituals for welcoming babies and honoring them throughout their childhood are believed to build children's self-esteem and help them know how much they are cherished. There are three welcoming rituals: a newborn ceremony, a naming ceremony at forty-two days, and the *Tiga Bulan* ceremony when a baby is three months of age. The *Tiga Bulan* (literally meaning three moons) is an elaborate four-hour ritual in which family members pray for the baby's health and long life while a priest blesses the parents, baby, and a spot on the earth where the baby's feet are first touched to the ground. Before this ceremony, during the first three months of life, a baby is considered "of the heavens" and is constantly held in someone's arms. At the conclusion of this ceremony, the baby is considered "of the earth." At this point, the baby can be put down, "out of arms," but I have rarely seen a Balinese infant or toddler not being held or closely watched. Babies are never put in another room or left alone; they are always within eyesight of at least one or more loving family members (see photo 5).

Every six lunar months (rather than our yearly birthdays) there is a special *Oton,* ceremony. The child's mother at this time returns to the coconut tree under which the baby's placenta was buried with offerings and special prayers for her child to have a long and healthy life. Offerings are also made here when the child is ill or needs special protection. A baby's umbilical cord, however, is never buried with the placenta. It is, instead, dried and ground into a powder that is kept as treasured medicine for that child. A Balinese baby wears a necklace on which hangs a small silver box containing some of this powder. If someone caring for the baby believes he may be getting ill, some of the powder is immediately mixed with sterile water and fed to the baby. This umbilical powder seems to have special immune protection for that particular person and is used throughout his life. (Use of the umbilical cord as medicine is also done in Japan, where each baby's dried cord is kept in a separate cedar box to be used for that particular person.) In Bali, if a baby is stillborn or later dies, the period of mourning is expected to be more intense and last much longer than for the loss of any other family member, "because babies are just so very special."

When I ask the Balinese what their goals are as parents, the answer is: "To help my children become the best at who they were meant to be." Believing that each child is born with special gifts, Balinese parents encourage their children to develop those talents to become as self-actualized as possible. If parents try to control, manipulate, or change a child in any way, they are considered to be failing as parents, and everyone in the village will let them know. Each child is equally respected regardless of his gift or role in the family—an artist, musician, accountant, cook, housekeeper, gardener, etc.—as long as he is being true to who he is meant to be.

Balinese are exceptionally egalitarian with both men and women in equal jobs and positions of respect. Men in Bali are very involved in caring for their children, with nurturing being valued more by Balinese men than macho behavior (see photo 6). While breastfeeding mothers are expected to remain close by their infants, the fathers often are seen holding, wearing, and comforting their babies to give the mothers a break and to develop their own close relationships. When the baby gets older and mom is working, it is common for men to spend the day with their toddlers and young children, delighting in playing with and taking care of them. Fathers are observed giving lots of affection to their children; it is common to see sons in their preteen years still sitting on their dad's lap and teenagers sitting next to their fathers with his arm around them (see photo 7).

Whenever a child is ill, both parents are involved, taking turns round the clock caring for the child until she is well again. As Balinese become adolescents, I have never observed the kind of animosity that typically exists between teens and parents in the US. Instead, Balinese adolescents are given respect as they take more responsibility for helping the family and are welcomed as adults.

Young boys in Bali seem observably calmer than their age-mates in the US. They exhibit less hyperactive and aggressive behaviors. Although they can be wild and playful, they often sit quietly, just watching, talking, and relaxing with friends. It is also common to find older boys playing with and caring for younger children.

In terms of discipline, the Balinese assume that since all children are born with "goodness inside," if a parent can just help the child "listen inside," the child will make good decisions. When the Balinese first explained this to me, the idea of disciplining by just helping a toddler listen inside didn't seem reasonable. I became convinced, however, after watching an example of this type of parenting. One day while visiting a Balinese family, I gave a balloon to a little two-year-old girl. She was happily playing with it until her two-and-a-half-year-old male cousin entered and snatched it away. The girl started to cry. The little boy's mother leaned down and quietly asked him, "Did you want to make your cousin cry?" He shook his head. Mom then asked, "Can you think of something that will make her happy again?" The little boy looked down at the balloon in his hands, then ran over and handed it to his cousin. All the family members sitting around praised the mom, and told the little boy how clever he was. I was extremely impressed with how quickly and gently it had been resolved. In less than one minute, a positive "win-win" situation had been created for each of them! I imagined how that might have been handled "back home." It would most likely have ended up with the boy feeling shamed, resentful, and angry, rather than being reinforced as clever, generous, and kind. I began wondering how this type of discipline would work in other situations.

Upon returning to the States, I soon had an opportunity to try out this method of introspective discipline. My daughter, Emily, was just entering middle school. After a few days, she came home and was swearing terribly. I was shocked since I had never heard her talk this way before and asked what was going on. She replied, "All the kids in middle school talk this way." I thought for a moment—how would the Balinese handle this? Turning to Emily, I calmly replied, "I didn't realize that was the kind of person you were inside," then added, "you are practicing the type of woman you'll be, so it is important to decide if that's how you really want to sound." She instantly stopped swearing.

While living with the Balinese, I had much opportunity to interview villagers about parenting. Wayan Ratna, a young mother who speaks English well, was born to a Balinese mother and an Australian father and has lived in both countries. Ratna blends the two cultures into her life in Bali and does not believe that either one has all the answers. She does like, however, the way the Balinese pay so much attention to the children and believes that "even small amounts of touch and talk are big for children." She explained that in Bali the babies really feel loved and respected, adding, "The ways we care about the babies really makes a lot of difference. If the parents teach them in more caring ways, the children will grow more in caring ways."[23]

Ketut Karta, an internationally-known artist, is a leader in the village of Penestanan, Bali. Karta strongly believes that it is important for all parents, including dads, to spend at least fifty percent of their time with their children. He stated that, "If people get lucky with their business, then they sometimes forget about their children—but most important is giving love to your children. If our children get healthy, happy, and feel loved that's better than money."[24] The Balinese think childhood should be filled with fun and everyone seems to love playing with the kids.

Nyoman Gandri is the mother of two boys. She reminded me of the gender-equality shared by Balinese couples when she explained, "My husband helps with everything in our house—cooking, washing, and making ceremonies."[25] About ten years ago, Nyoman told me a story that really concerned the Balinese villagers:

> A mother from the US was visiting Bali for a few months with her nine-month-old son and hired Nyoman's sister Ketut to help care for the little boy. Each morning the mom left her son for most of the day. The baby didn't cry when his mom would leave, but after a few weeks, the baby started crying when Ketut left. The mom then told Ketut that she shouldn't hold the baby so much because it was clearly making him less independent, and that it wasn't the "American way." Villagers were shocked, and concerned that Americans are not giving babies enough nurturing. She then added, "I think the baby likes the Balinese way better, because we have heard that even years later whenever the little boy cries, he calls for Ketut."[26]

When I asked my "Balinese son," Made Narok, why he thought Balinese parents were so kind to their children, he laughingly answered, "Parents must be very good to their children since their children will be taking care of them when they are old."[27] The Balinese know that how we care for our children in their younger years is directly related to how we will be cared for in our elder years (see photo 8).

One of the most valuable parenting practices I have learned from watching peaceful parents is the importance of building and protecting the relationship with your child and when you feel disconnected, doing your best to reconnect as soon as possible. Parenting in the context of a close relationship is not only more joyful, but results in cooperative, kind children and happy families.

## A Culture Striving to Become Peaceful

### Japanese

In 2002, our family took a trip to Japan in the wake of the September 11, 2001 terrorist attack on the United States. Due to our newly-felt national grief and vulnerability, we wanted to visit Hiroshima and pay our respects to Japanese people who had lost their lives, loved ones, and health due to the atomic bombing by the US during World War II. We did not know until this journey that after WWII, the people of Japan had made a national commitment to never again be part of another war. Much controversy by the Japanese people has accompanied a recent July 1, 2014 reinterpretation of Article 9 of the Japanese Constitution, which is now permitting military forces to be used for self-defense. [28] It is heartwarming to know that for sixty-nine years, that nation made a significant attempt to heal from their painful past and create a more peaceful future. In spite of this newly-initiated governmental policy, hopefully the long-held commitment to nonviolence by the Japanese people will continue.

Our family felt great remorse when we visited the Hiroshima memorial to over one hundred fifty thousand civilians, a large percentage of them children, who died from the US nuclear bombing on August 6, 1945. Obviously Americans, we wondered how we would be received by the people of Hiroshima. An experience we will always remember helped us truly believe that compassion can heal human hearts and reconciliation is possible.

Early one morning we sat in the Peace Park outside the Memorial Museum, gathering our courage to enter and face displays of the most horrendous destruction ever unleashed on humankind. Suddenly, a very frail older Japanese woman who most likely had lived through that horrific event approached us. In broken English, she inquired if we were

Americans. I quickly answered, "Yes, we are here to offer our heartfelt apology to your people who have suffered and died." With tears in her eyes, she told us that she very rarely sees Americans there, and asked if she could bless us. After giving our shocked consents, the old woman raised her wrinkled arms and held her hands for a very long time above each of our heads. Tears rolled down all of our faces, as a sacred feeling of the oneness in humanity washed over us along with a blossoming of hope that perhaps it may be possible for people to find a way to coexist peacefully on this planet.

To promote the Japanese people's commitment to creating a nonviolent society, one of the high priorities for the Japanese government has been support of new parents and encouragement for them to spend much time nurturing their infants. Growing a generation of children who are more compassionate seems to have been their goal.

In Japan, after childbirth a mother is kept in the hospital with round-the-clock lactation help until breastfeeding is well established. Upon returning home, the baby is not taken out in public for at least four weeks. The new mom and infant spend all their time together during this period of bonding, while the mom's own mom usually cares for the house and any older children. Friends and family members bring food and leave it on the doorstep, but do not enter the house so as not to interrupt this important stage of maternal attachment.

All Japanese mothers are given an optional *one-year paid* maternity leave and encouraged to continue breastfeeding throughout the baby's first year. The government provides the mother with monthly income during that entire year and employers are required to return the mother's job to her at any time up to the baby's first birthday. Each new mom is also invited to join a government-funded mothers' support group lasting throughout the baby's first year. The group provides weekly activities for new moms living near each other, who have babies within two to three months of each other. When the year ends, the mothers are encouraged to continue meeting on their own with their support group.[29]

When in Tokyo, I had the pleasure of interviewing Naho Kikuchi, a counselor at an international school. Naho, the mother of two children, talked about being very thankful for her government's paid maternity leave. She described how wonderful spending the first year at home with her daughter had been for their relationship. Naho had stayed home only four months after the birth of her first child and besides finding it difficult to continue breastfeeding, she wishes that she would have stayed home longer with him.[30] Additional information from this interview will be shared in upcoming chapters.

## Other Cultures Shaped My Own Mothering

Within weeks after returning from the extended travel adventure in Central and South America, I became pregnant with our firstborn son, Shane. Having observed parenting practices that stirred a deep inner knowing of how babies should be nurtured, I knew that I could not parent in the traditional American fashion promoted at the time. Understanding that this decision would require repeated defending of my strangely unorthodox mothering behaviors, I embarked on the most important journey in my life. I chose a newly-opened birthing clinic with a nurse midwife who supported a birthing experience that at the time was revolutionary: completely natural birth (extremely rare), my husband being fully involved (just becoming acceptable), and keeping the baby always with me (unheard of).

I was strongly committed to exclusive breastfeeding, though this was uncommon during the mid-seventies. Breasts were frequently exposed in media sources of the day, but North Americans seemed to have lost sight of their principal purpose—to feed babies. Infants were typically fed formula and kept on an every-four-hour feeding schedule. Within the first few days of my breastfeeding Shane whenever he wanted to nurse, my husband questioned whether I should be nursing our newborn again after just an hour had passed. I responded with deep instinctual knowing, "Well, I never saw a Bolivian mother look at a clock before putting her baby to the breast."

I wore Shane in a front pack whenever possible and secretly bed-shared with him, something that was medically taboo in the US because it was espoused as being physically dangerous and emotionally damaging.

There were many raised eyebrows and furled brows in my family and community concerning how I, a specialist in child development, was raising my son. To the surprise of everyone, my greatest advocate was my dear ninety-year-old grandmother who had ancient wisdom of her own. One day, she leaned close to my ear and quietly whispered, "You just keep giving Shane as much love as you can while he is young, and one day he'll take care of you, because he'll know how to love." Then she pulled back, stood tall, and confidently stated, "It isn't just a coincidence that I'm not in a nursing home!" Relieved to have Grandma Dina's validation, I gave Shane as much love as I could, and when he became a very happy, content, and kind little boy, many who questioned my mothering became intrigued.

# CHAPTER 2

# Attachment

*Feelings of love and gratitude arise directly and spontaneously*
*in a baby, in response to love and care . . .*
—Melanie Klein

Attachment for human infants is a matter of life or death. Born completely helpless, an infant's basic survival depends on continuing a close relationship with his mother or someone who can provide food and care for all his needs. Humans appear to be born only halfway through their gestation. All other mammals can crawl to a food source within days or weeks after birth, but it takes a human infant another nine months. Anthropologists believe that when our ancestors began to walk upright, the structure of the pelvic area began to change in order to make walking easier. Birth was initially not a problem because at that time our brains were small and could easily slip through the narrowing pelvic bones. Walking on two legs, however, suddenly made hands available to do so many new things that it caused our brains to began growing. In the past 1.5 million years, human brains have developed into the largest brains relative to body size of any living mammal.[1] If babies were born truly "full term," their heads would no longer fit through the birth canal. So, as brains grew, babies began to be born earlier and earlier. Currently, infants are born at forty weeks of gestation and need constant care with readily available food for at least another forty weeks until they can crawl and feed themselves. In terms of early development, our infants are much like baby kangaroos, which need to be continually carried and fed. Their immaturity requires a closely committed attachment for survival, a devoted caregiver willing to meet all of their needs during this critical "second half of gestation." Since the largest growth of the human brain now takes place after birth, a baby who has someone who delights in providing consistent nurturing care helps the baby develop a brain wired with feelings of security, self-worth,

19

and trust in relationships, this becomes the foundation of that child's personality.

## Parenting by Other Primates

From an evolutionary standpoint, it is interesting not only to observe parenting practices of human cultures, but also to consider how our closest living nonhuman relatives attempt to meet the needs of their infants. I have spent time watching bands of macaque monkeys in a Balinese monkey forest, as well as langur monkeys in the Himalayan areas of India and Nepal. Parenting by these primates is more instinctual, focused on meeting the actual needs of their babies without being influenced by popular beliefs and cultures.

The macaques are considered "mono-bonders," meaning there is a single female, usually the mother, to whom an infant becomes attached.[2] Macaque mothers are very attentive and nurturing to their own infants, constantly "wearing" their babies and nursing them "at will" for one to two years. Even while mothers are walking or climbing, it is common to see the babies riding on their mother's back or dangling under their chests, clutching tightly to their mom's body and suckling. Baby monkeys, while awake or asleep, accompany their mother in all of her daily activities. Although macaque mothers live in groups, offering each other social support, they do not like sharing their babies. When macaques get together, babies play together and mothers groom each other, but there is little interaction among mothers toward infants who are not their own. This is similar to our human mothering behavior in current Western cultures. When others ask to hold the baby, this doesn't usually mean they are willing to take responsibility for all of the baby's needs. More often than not, the baby is instantly returned to his mother as soon as he becomes uncomfortable.

In comparison to the macaques, the langurs are referred to as "cooperative breeders." Langur mothers trust their close relatives to care for their babies to up to fifty percent of the daytime hours.[3] Young females are especially eager to care for the babies. It gives them practice in caregiving before becoming mothers themselves.[4]

## Balinese Infant Sharing

During an Independence Day celebration in Bali, I followed a baby around for an hour. She spent approximately:

- 10 minutes with her mom
- 20 minutes with her dad's dad
- 15 minutes with mom's cousin
- 10 minutes with dad's brother

When she started missing her mom . . .

- She was given back to mom for about 5 minutes until the next person asked to hold her.

This mom had her baby in her arms only about 15 minutes during the entire hour. In an infant-sharing culture, it is clearly easier for a new mother to have both personal freedom and a close, loving attachment with her infant.

This type of "infant sharing" is similar to what happens in human cultures such as the Balinese, who depend on direct assistance from family members in caring for their youngsters. The "infant sharing" Balinese continually pass their babies from one person to another. Holding a baby is an honor in Bali, so mothers get incredible hands-on support. This constantly available caregiving makes it easier for mothers to meet the intense needs of their infants without becoming overwhelmed and exhausted.

## Importance of Parental Attachment

In the 1950s, during the era in which infant formula was believed to be healthier than breast milk, Harry Harlow, an experimental psychologist, was using rhesus monkeys for his research studies. Attempting to decrease infant mortality in his research subjects, the baby monkeys were removed from their mothers soon after birth and placed in cages where they could be bottle-fed with formula enriched with iron and vitamin supplements. Much to Harlow's surprise, the caged infants' health began to deteriorate, and infant mortality increased. Another observation was that the bottle-fed babies raised alone, rather than becoming more independent, actually exhibited high levels of anxiety. Instead of playing and exploring like mother-raised babies, they clung to their own bodies and compulsively rocked back and forth, similar to emotionally deprived human children raised in institutions. When Harlow put soft terry cloth-covered cones in the cages, the lonely infants desperately would cling to this soft substitute mother, and their self-hugging repetitive rocking decreased.

Harlow began to question why a mother seemed to be so important for normal development. Many had previously believed that infants were only attached to their mothers due to their ability to feed the babies. Further research clearly showed that an infant monkey actually preferred a soft terry cloth "mom" without any food to a plain wire "mom" with a protruding nipple from which they could constantly feed. Babies only used the wire "moms" for eating, while the remainder of the time was spent frantically clinging to the cuddlier terry cloth "moms" for comfort. When all of these maternally deprived infants later had their own babies, they were terrible at mothering. In fact, they were so inadequate that their babies wouldn't have even survived if Harlow hadn't arranged for the babies to be hand-fed. Generations of neglect and abuse cannot continue in the wild, because the offspring do not survive.[5] In human families, however, cycles of child neglect and abuse are continually passed to future generations, unless there is awareness of the damage being done and a strong determination to change it.

A British psychologist, John Bowlby, the pioneer of attachment theory in the 1950s, explained that a newborn human instinctively needs to feel attached to a caregiver in order to survive. Bowlby believed, "the infant and young child should experience a warm, intimate, and continuous relationship with his mother (or permanent mother substitute) in which both find satisfaction and enjoyment."[6] He also concluded that as the baby matures, this close attachment helps ensure that as a toddler, he will stick close by that parent in times of danger.[7] In fact, with human children close parental attachments are necessary to meet all major needs during their first *eighteen years* of life.

A Canadian psychologist, Mary Ainsworth, worked in John Bowlby's London clinic in the 1950s and became interested in the role of mother-infant attachment. Attachment at that time was so misunderstood that hospitals did not even allow parents to visit their sick children. When parents left after visiting hours, the children cried and were seriously distressed. When parents did not visit, the children were much quieter and easier to manage. It was, therefore, believed to be better for children to have parents drop them off and not visit them at all throughout their hospital stays. Bowlby and Ainsworth were able to radically change hospital policies by showing that when children endured painful, frightening medical interventions without parents present, the children didn't cry because they went from being distressed, to depressed, to detached. When these children later returned home, they had great difficulty reattaching to their parents because their basic trust had been so undermined. Bowlby and Ainsworth convinced others that crying was a positive sign of secure attachment and should be respected, without attempts to eliminate it.[8]

Dr. Ainsworth broadened her research on maternal attachment by studying mother-infant relationships in both Africa and the US. She consistently found that (1) mothers who responded quickly to their babies had secure attachments that resulted in infants who cried less and were easily comforted, (2) mothers who gave their babies attention but seemed to misread their babies' cues had babies who cried a lot, and (3) mothers who were unresponsive to their babies, often leaving them alone, had babies who appeared to shut down, not even caring if their mothers were in the room.[9]

These revolutionary findings were in direct contradiction to the popularly held Western cultural belief that if crying babies were responded to quickly, they would be "spoiled" and end up becoming whiny, demanding toddlers. Babies are damaged when they don't get enough consistent attention and sensitive nurturing. Another misunderstood concept is that babies who receive too much nurturing won't become independent or learn to "self-calm." Again, the opposite is true. Independence comes from security, and security comes from having your needs consistently met when you are dependent on others. Ainsworth concluded,

"Infants whose mothers have given them relatively tender and affection- ate holding in the earliest months of life are content with surprisingly little physical contact by the end of the first year ... although they enjoy being held, when put down they are happy to move off into independent exploratory play."[10]

For the first year and a half, infants have physical and emotional needs that they can't meet on their own. They become attached to dependable caregivers who are warm, sensitive, and try to understand and satisfy those needs. As babies become mobile, they use these attachment figures as secure bases from which they can explore their worlds, knowing they will be welcomed and cared for when they return. While infants' brains are not developed enough to learn appropriate behaviors, by about eigh- teen months toddlers are able to begin learning what is socially acceptable and at that point need clear expectations and limit setting. Early close attachments make limit setting much easier, because toddlers delight in pleasing the person to whom they feel a close warm relationship.

The foundation for a positive lifelong parent-child relationship begins with a parent's desire to fulfill her infant's needs for physical and emo- tional closeness during the first eighteen months of life. Six decades of research have consistently shown how critically important attachment is in being able to feel secure and trust in relationships. Parenting practices that focus on creating intimate loving attachments can help infants not only survive, but thrive.

## The Magical First Hour

While parental attachment in humans usually begins at some point during the pregnancy, the ninety minutes immediately following birth is hormonally primed to be the most powerful period of attachment between parents and their infants. The newborn has just gone through childbirth, one of life's most traumatic challenges, but will become calm if she remains within a three-foot radius of her mother. An infant removed from the mother usually begins screaming, experiencing extreme anxiety, with increased levels of cortisol (a hormone released during severe stress) of up to ten times the normal level.[11]

If a newborn is kept close to her mother and was not overly medicated during the birth, she will enter into a calm "quiet alert state" during this first face-to-face meeting. Especially interested in faces, she will gaze into the eyes of whoever is holding her. An infant can recognize her mother's smell and voice, as well as the voice of her father or others she has heard while in the womb. All of the baby's energy is channeled into looking, listening, and connecting.[12] Attachment between mother, father, and baby is deeply assisted by skin-to-skin contact during this eye-gazing period and is described by parents as a most joyful time of "falling in love" with their baby. The hormones oxytocin and prolactin, released in the mother's and father's brains, assist in making this time especially blissful. Research has shown that mothers who have this early period of bonding with their newborns continue later to engage in more affectional maternal behaviors such as close holding, hugging, kissing, fondling, vocalizing, eye to eye contact, and smiling at their infants.[13]

When an unmedicated infant is placed on her mom's belly immediately after birth, she has an instinctive ability to crawl up to a breast, find the nipple, self-attach, and begin suckling, all within the first fifty-five minutes.[14] The UNICEF/World Health Organization's Baby-Friendly Hospital Initiative now requires that infants be put skin-to-skin with their mothers and left undisturbed for at least the first hour, stating that "helping mothers to initiate breastfeeding within one hour after birth" is one of the ten most important steps to successful initiation and continuation of breastfeeding.[15]

Prolactin is a wonderful "parenting hormone" that stimulates relaxation, patience, protection, nurturing behavior, and attachment. The name prolactin, referring to "pro-lactation," is a hormone clearly associated with breastfeeding mothers. Less known is the fact that prolactin is also present in males. Primate studies have found that male tamarin monkeys have increased levels of prolactin right after their mates give birth and when the males are in close proximity to babies and pregnant or lactating mothers. Prolactin is five times higher in male marmoset monkeys that carry around their offspring.[16] Research suggests that hormones in a human father are also affected by his mate's pregnancy and when he is intimately involved in the birthing experience. The hormones prolactin, vasopressin, and oxytocin can all increase in men at the time of their baby's birth. These hormones promote attachment, protection, love, loyalty, commitment, and caring in the new father.[17] Perhaps this is why Balinese men, who spend a great deal of time directly taking care of their young children, are also very gentle and nurturing with them. We are seeing an increase in nurturing behaviors among those fathers in developed countries who are directly involved in caring for their infants.

## Father's Role After Birth

The complete dependence of newborns makes forming a securely attached relationship with a vigilant caregiver critical. In theory, this can be anyone, however, a human infant has a primal desire for this first relationship outside the womb to be a continuation of the relationship with his mother that began and developed over nine months within the womb. Infants long to feel the continuance of this original maternal attachment particularly during the "second half of gestation" that occurs in the first nine months outside of the womb.

Noticeable in my work with children and adults who have lost birth mothers due to death, abandonment, or adoption, even when loving fathers, grandparents, or adoptive parents have raised them, is that there is a deep unsettled angst caused by the early maternal loss. We know that not all babies will be welcomed by their birth mothers, but it seems necessary for us to accept that this situation causes significant distress. When a mother-infant relationship is severed, the baby experiences a profound sense of loss that has some long-lasting consequences.

A breastfeeding mother and infant have an especially close relationship assisted by the nurturing hormones stimulated in each of them and the synchronicity of how their bodies continue to be intimately interconnected. While a loving father can offer every type of comfort to his baby except for breastfeeding, the infant will often want to be with his mother because of the relief and refuge that nursing provides as the immature brain seeks to maintain its first attachment. It is important for dads to understand this vital breastfeeding bond, which provides their babies with not only the best nutrition possible, but also a strong foundation of emotional security.

Dads can become confused about their role during the first nine months of intense dependency on the mother. Certain dads feel left out, jealous, or even resentful of the close breastfeeding relationship. Patrick Houser, a leader in the promotion of early involved fathering says, "Some fathers think less is best and the sooner I get *my breasts*, and my wife back, the better."[18] Other dads will compete with the new mother, wanting the baby to pay as much attention to him. While attached dads' roles during their babies' first year of life can be perplexing, in peaceful cultures it is more clearly understood.

A Tibetan father is expected to take over the household chores while giving the baby's mother lots of extra nurturing and encouraging her to get as much sleep as possible so she is able to offer their newborn a warm, securely-attached beginning. The foundation for a close father-baby bond begins at the beginning with the father offering as much care of the baby as possible, and supporting the baby to be with his mother when the baby wants her. The rewards from a dad's early attachment with his infant are often experienced more directly after the nine-month-old baby emerges from the "second half of gestation" and begins delighting more in being with his father who was supportive of the mother-baby bond. This certainly does not mean that a father should retreat to only the protector-provider role of past generations, but instead that he should stay as involved as possible in the hands-on caregiving of his baby, as explained in Jack Heinowitz's book, *Fathering Right from the Start: Straight Talk about Pregnancy, Birth, and Beyond.*[19] Loving care by a new father during these early months after birth can include skin-to-skin contact, wearing the baby in a sling, comforting, changing diapers, playing, talking, singing, dancing, etc., all of which become the foundation of a strong securely-attached father-infant relationship. The challenge for new moms is to support dads in their involvement with the baby, realizing that even though dads may do things differently, what matters most is that they are doing them. Moms often inadvertently sabotage dads' caregiving of the baby by believing that as moms, they know the best way to do everything related to their babies' care. Accepting that babies can benefit from having things done in more than one way will go a long way in encouraging more involvement and cooperation from dads.

During past generations in the US, fathers were minimally involved in the direct care of their babies. Before the 1970s, dads were not even allowed to be part of their own babies' birthing experiences! The decade following the American women's liberation movement created much change for both genders. Men were not only welcomed into the delivery rooms, but as women began having careers outside the home, dads were expected to be much more involved in the direct care of their children. Some of those fathers were very conflicted about these new expectations, and resentments often arose between the parents when caregiving the children clashed with dads' career advancements or providing financially for their families. Conflict was also felt by mothers who wanted to be home with their infants while also dreaming of having a satisfying career. The resulting divorce rate in the US became one of the highest in the world. All of this angst was probably a natural part of the evolution that takes place when a society strives for such changes in gender equality.

Fathers of the current generation raised by dads who were hands-on caregivers, seem much more open to embracing their roles as nurturers. Patrick Houser believes that nurturing hormones stimulated when dads are more involved with their babies have resulted in an enhancement of "bonding, attachment, protection, loyalty, commitment, and caring" in new fathers."[20] In Houser's article, "The Science of Father Love," printed in a 2011 newsletter of the Association for Prenatal and Perinatal Psychology and Health, he claims that when men's nurturing instincts and hormones were awakened, our society became destined to have a different future. Houser states that, "Children have led fathers through the doorway of tenderness and we have all entered a new era." Fathers who are attached to their infants from the beginning continue to be more involved with their toddlers. In one-third of parent-caregiver households with young children, the at-home parent is now the father.[21]

Many developed countries have government-financed support for paid parental leave of more than one year. In those countries, the mother usually spends most of the first year with the baby, but a few weeks to months of the leave are reserved just for fathers, with the second and third years often shared between the parents. One of my greatest hopes is that American society will someday have such governmental support for new parents. This could help babies significantly to get the early nurturing they need, while reducing parental stress and increasing marital satisfaction. I saw a great bumper sticker recently, which read, "Men who change diapers change the world."

## Maternal Ambivalence

Even though females are hormonally "wired" to form intimate relationships and feel nurturing toward their infants, many human mothers experience ambivalence rather than motherly love; this is uncommon among other primates. Anthropologist Sarah Blaffer Hrdy has found that the psychological struggle between the equally strong desires for personal freedom and maternal attachment can produce a conflict for human mothers.[22] The American women's movement suddenly created much independence for women, including opportunities for jobs outside the home, degrees in higher education, and positions of professional respect. Previous generations had observed a high percentage of mothers feeling unhappily trapped as "housewives," bound exclusively to the care of their homes, husbands, and children. Many of those mothers resented not having the freedom to actualize their own abilities and ambitions.

Various conditions in a mother's life influence how nurturing she will be to her baby. If a woman believes she will have to sacrifice too many of her own needs, she tends to resist closely attaching to her infant. It is not just having a parent available that is critical, but one that enjoys providing the physical and emotional nurturing the baby needs. What mothers require in order to form such close, loving relationships with their newborns is emotional, financial, and hands-on support from their partners, extended families, and community as is provided in most indigenous cultures and in many other developed countries.

Naho Kikuchi in Japan stated that what is most important in becoming a good mother is to feel supported by your own mother, other older women, and close friends who are mothers. She explained that when a woman has a baby in Japan, it is culturally expected that her own mother will help her daughter become a successful mother. When a woman is about to give birth, she usually goes to her own parents' home and the baby is born in their city. The baby's father is involved in the birth, but returns to the couples' home soon after in order to work. The new mother typically stays with her parents for the month following childbirth. If the maternal grandmother is not available to help out, other members of the mother's family will care for the new mom and baby.[23]

As one of those "women's libbers" protesting in the early 1970s, I'll be forever thankful for all the changes that helped me achieve my personal and professional goals. My generation benefited greatly from increased opportunities and enjoyed the wealth produced by two-income families. Another factor that enabled mothers to be away from their infants for increasingly extended periods was that by the early 1970s, over seventy-five percent of babies in the US were fed almost entirely with commercially-produced infant formulas.[24] In retrospect we have come to realize that our baby-boomer generation was unaware of how important maternal nurturing was to our newborns. The mental health crises among children, along with recent research findings on early brain development, are forcing us to reevaluate some of these parenting practices. Currently in the US, babies commonly have some form of childcare by an unrelated adult for more than eight hours a day from the time they are only twelve weeks of age.

Without pointing fingers of blame, it is tugging at our heartstrings to realize that young children have not been getting the time, attention,

---

**Maternal ambivalence is not just a recent condition.**

In France in the late 1700s, 95% of urban infants were sent to rural areas to be wet-nursed by strangers who were paid for this service. French mothers felt they would lose too much of their identities, and abilities to work outside the home if they nursed their own babies. Early mothering was not considered of great consequence to children's development, resulting in many mothers not even seeing their infants for the entire first year of their lives.[25]

---

or nurturance they require to be as physically or emotionally healthy as possible. Even though parents are increasingly stressed "to the max" trying to meet obligations of careers, homes, finances, and care for their children, it appears that their infants and toddlers are being seriously shortchanged.

Although increased educational and professional opportunities allow new mothers more autonomy, the basic needs of babies have not changed. The primary love-bond formed in the first year provides the foundation for a child's ability to feel self-worth and trust in relationships.[25] During the next two years, toddlers develop a conscience, begin to understand expectations, gain some self-control, and learn how to get along with others. Many researchers are calling these first three years the most important "one thousand days" of a person's life.

While most mothers do not want to return to the discontent of previous generations who felt trapped without choices, they definitely want to meet their young children's needs. It is important for new parents to understand that infants and toddlers' needs for nurturing do not mean mothers must give up their careers and embrace the "housewife" category of past generations. The period needed to create a trusting foundation, optimize brain development, and learn to be self-disciplined is about three years. We willingly spend a few years of our lives training for a new career, at least two years in an apprenticeship or getting an associate's degree, four years for a bachelor's degree, and many more years earning advanced degrees. Isn't a period of one to three years actually a small amount of time to devote to raising an emotionally healthy child? When parents spend these first few years building healthy children, they spend much less time and money later trying to fix behavior problems that may develop. When I was in Bhutan, I saw a poster on the wall that sums it up well: "It is much easier to build a child than to repair an adult."

## Necessity of Social Support

For a new mother to form a loving attachment to her newborn, she, herself, must feel loved, cared for, and supported. In the words of Subonfu Somé, a brilliant cross-cultural educator from West Africa, "It takes a village to raise a child and a community to keep parents sane."[27] A major factor in a mother's success during pregnancy, birth, and breastfeeding is the quality of care she receives from the baby's father.[28] Along with having support from her partner, extended family, friends, employer, and government programs, women are also in need of social support from other women.

A study conducted in the year 2000 investigated ways that women deal with stress.[29] Previous studies, which described the reaction to stress as an adrenalin driven "fight-or-flight" response, had used only male subjects. This recent more thorough "Tend and Befriend Study" revealed an important difference between males and females in terms of their response to stress. When under stress, men produce a high level of testosterone, which leads to a "fight-or-flight" response. But, it is hypothesized that in women, the hormone oxytocin is released during stress to help buffer the fight-or-flight response. Oxytocin, one of the "love hormones," creates a desire for connection with others. Considering the specific roles of men and women in ancient times, a difference in stress-related brain chemistry makes sense. When there were threats to the clan, men were required to go fight the danger, while women needed to help each other quiet the children and keep them safe. We all know that when women are under stress, the first thing they often do is grab the phone and call another woman who can listen and offer support. As women engage in this "tending and befriending" behavior, it appears that even more oxytocin is released, further reducing stress and increasing calmness. Many studies have found that close friendships between women not only help them cope with stressful events, but that women who reach out to other women for support have lower blood pressure, reduced cholesterol, and tend to live longer.[30]

Humans are "pack or clan animals," extremely reliant on the support of a trusted group.[31] We are much more like wolves than cougars, and like the "lone wolf," we do not survive if we become too independent or isolated. While the stated goal of most American parents is that their children become "independent," this contradicts with our fundamental human need for close interdependent relationships. Even the most adventurous pioneers came over the Rocky Mountains in large wagon trains, knowing that their basic survival depended on sharing and caring for each other. They formed close supportive relationships and worked cooperatively to built houses, barns, and communities. People are again realizing that rebuilding connections to our extended families and recreating community along with helping our children learn to become "interdependent" could help us all have happier, healthier lives.

A loving relationship between a baby and her parents is the foundation for the child becoming a healthy person. Our need for connection is so strong that humans truly need love more than we even need food or water. Babies who are given adequate food, but not lovingly nurtured can fail to gain weight, and even die. These babies' diagnosis is merely "failure to thrive."

Watching youngsters in peaceful cultures flourish when being treated with unconditional love and respect by all the adults in their village has been very heartwarming. Children who are treated with affection feel lovable, and are then able to be loving. While this may sound simplistic, love *is* the guiding force of happiness in human beings. Just think of what people will do for love. People will kill for love, will kill themselves if they feel unloved, and will even kill the person they love most if that person doesn't love them back. Even as adults, feeling loved radically changes our basic feelings of well-being. We all know how joyful it feels to be cherished by others and how painful it is to feel unimportant, disregarded, or discarded.

## Extended Family Support in Bali

Balinese live in extended family compounds with a communally shared courtyard that contains the kitchen, eating, and living area. Individual sleeping rooms (one for each nuclear family) surround the courtyard. When a boy marries, his wife will leave her own family and go live with her husband's family. This extended family living means that the children are always being cared for and played with by lots of family members of all ages. Balinese believe that constant nurturing grows loving children.

The current generation of young parents in the US is becoming aware of the importance of extended family and community support for raising healthy and happy children. The previous generation was more individually focused and attempted to parent in isolated nuclear or single parent families. Extremely high levels of depression and anxiety even in our children indicate that this was not successful. Young parents who don't have extended family involvement are beginning to develop relationships with other new parents and create supportive "villages" to help each other in the ominous and extremely rewarding job of raising emotionally healthy children.

# CHAPTER 3

# Mindful Parenting of Infants

*I carry your heart with me. I carry it in my heart.*
*I am never without it. Anywhere I go, you go, my dear.*
—E. E. Cummings

Mindful Parenting is my own blend of parenting practices which has evolved over four decades of studying child development, observing parenting throughout the world, helping clients heal from their childhood traumas, and experimenting with these techniques as a mother with my own son and daughter. Mindful Parenting of infants involves being aware, engaged, and responsive to your baby's needs, with the ultimate goal of creating a closely attached relationship. Mindful Parenting incorporates parenting practices from peaceful cultures that welcome newborns with elaborate rituals and extensive nurturing, guaranteeing that infants feel cherished, and unconditionally loved.

## Practices that Increase Attachment

- Skin-to-Skin Contact
- Breastfeeding
- Wearing Babies
- Co-Sleeping
- Affection
- Listening
- Responding
- Singing
- Playing
- Close Proximity

## Global Practices that Increase Attachment

Parenting practices I have observed throughout the world that create close, mutually-secure attachments are: skin-to-skin contact, breastfeeding, wearing babies, co-sleeping, affection, listening, responding, singing, playing, and close proximity. Attachment is promoted when parents engage in these practices as soon as their baby is born. When this is not possible, for instance in the case of a medical emergency or adoption, it is best if parents begin these practices as soon as they are able. Even with an older adopted toddler, adding as many of these ways to connect as you possibly can will increase the probability of creating a secure attachment.

### Skin-to-Skin Contact

There is much evidence supporting the importance of skin-to-skin contact, especially during the first ninety minutes after birth while the baby is in what is known as the "quiet alert stage." After going through the trauma of being squeezed through the birth canal and ejected into a completely foreign environment, the infant usually stops crying when held skin-to-skin, and gazes into his mother's eyes. Cradling the naked newborn on the mother's bare chest stimulates the hormone oxytocin in both the mom and baby, helping them fall in love with each other. When a newborn is welcomed in this way, he feels comforted by the familiar voice and smell of his mother in whom he has lived for nine months. This bodily contact and eye gazing ignites feelings of attachment as the baby begins his lifelong journey outside of the womb. Early skin-to-skin contact not only stimulates calm, loving feelings, but helps the baby in lots of other ways such as: regulating breathing, stabilizing the heart rate and body temperature, maintaining blood sugar level, being colonized by the mother's bacteria, scooting toward the breast, and rooting behavior that begins successful breastfeeding.[1]

In this first hour-and-a-half, it is also important for the baby to have skin-to-skin contact with his father, on his father's bare chest. The baby usually recognizes his father's voice and feels secure in his arms. "If a father is intimate with his child, especially through skin-to-skin contact, his own oxytocin production increases. Elevated oxytocin in a father is recognized as a key component in jump-starting and maintaining his nurturing instincts."[2] If the mother, due to a cesarean birth or other medical complications, is unable to have skin-to-skin contact during this ninety minute quiet alert stage, it is especially important for the father to hold the newborn on his naked chest during this time to offer reassurance, comfort, and love. At a cesarean birth I once attended, the father was told he wouldn't be able to hold the baby skin-to-skin because the hospital gown he had to wear was too tight. I quickly made my way down the hall to the gown cupboard and brought back a XXL gown, which offered plenty of extra room. When we requested that the frightened newborn be slipped between the gown and his father's bare chest, it worked perfectly. The anxiety of both dad and baby instantly melted away as the infant stopped screaming, quickly calming as he gazed into his father's tear-filled loving eyes.

While this skin-to-skin time is standard practice in cultures where babies are born at home or in birthing clinics, most hospitals have routine procedures that often compete with this important period of bonding. Parents birthing in a hospital can provide a written birth plan and should be firm in their resolve that this is *their* baby's birth, and they want to have the first ninety minutes for skin-to-skin holding without interruption unless there is a medical emergency. Even if a baby is born prematurely, skin-to-skin contact can help the baby stabilize, stay warm, and reduce his need for extra oxygen.

The Association for Prenatal and Perinatal Psychology and Health (APPPAH) has started a major international campaign to increase skin-to-skin contact as a primary method of easily and cheaply optimizing early attachment between parents and their newborns. APPPAH reports that one hour of skin-to-skin contact has been found to have long-term benefits for the baby and mother: (1) The baby in terms of breastfeeding, digestion, improved sleep, emotional attachment, and first-year developmental milestones. (2) The new mother in terms of improved postpartum recovery, emotional well-being, maternal attachment, and fewer complications with breastfeeding.[3]

Early skin-to-skin time is sometimes missed due to a medical emergency or in the case of adoption in which the adoptive parents are not present at the birth. While such a delay is not optimal, skin-to-skin contact can still be very helpful even when done at a later time. Affectionate touching, hugging, and cuddling by someone you trust directly stimulate loving feelings in all human relationships. Various ways to engage in skin-to-skin contact throughout infancy and toddlerhood are:

- Cradle the naked baby close to your bare chest while gently rocking him (perhaps with a soft blanket over his back).
- Lay with the baby on your chest for nap time (a diaper would help in this case).
- Take a bath with your baby and hold him close to you in the warm water.
- Hold baby skin-to-skin while singing or dancing with him.

Infant massage is another wonderfully pleasant age-old method of providing nurturing touch, relaxation, improved sleep, and close attachment between parents and their baby.[4]

I always encourage adoptive parents to spend some time skin-to-skin with their babies and toddlers to build feelings of closeness and attachment. It is particularly helpful with adopted children to go back and fill in some of the ways to promoting attachment that they missed, as long as you are sensitive to whether the child feels safe and is comfortable with such experiences. For some adopted children, it may take time for your touch to feel reassuring and pleasurable.

## Breastfeeding

Babies who are held skin-to-skin on their mother's chest during the first hour after birth have an instinctual ability to scoot up and latch on to their mother's breast. This act of suckling releases hormones that promote attachment, helping a mother and her infant feel closely interconnected. Swedish researchers found that if an infant's lips touched his mother's nipple within the first hour after birth, the mother kept that infant close to her one hundred minutes longer each day than mothers who didn't have this early suckling experience.[5]

While some mothers may choose not to breastfeed, they certainly deserve all available information before making this significant decision. Breast milk is perfectly designed for human infants and is without a doubt the best food possible, along with offering instant connection and comfort. Throughout the world, babies are breastfed whenever they are hungry, tired, or craving extra nurturing.

In Bali, Ratna told me she believed breastfeeding was most important for building a close relationship between a mother and her infant. She shared, "My young daughters were with me all the time. It makes the child closer to the mother and feel more sense of love." Ratna breastfed her older daughter for four years and the younger one for three years.[6] Nyoman, also from Bali, is a strong believer that breastfeeding helps a baby feel loved. "When drinking mother's milk the love feeling of the mother goes down into the baby." She breastfed her boys until they were five years of age.[7] As Dr. Mimi in Bhutan sat nursing her newborn son, she reported that Bhutanese babies are always breastfed for at least two years. She added that all babies were exclusively fed breast milk for the first four months before cereal was introduced, but added that she thought it should be a few months longer to avoid allergies and asthma. Even when Bhutanese mothers return to work, they are given a thirty-minute break every morning and afternoon during which their babies are brought to them to be nursed.[8]

It seems important to understand the relatively recent history of when and how Western mothers stopped breastfeeding their babies. In 1867, a German chemist developed the first infant formula, but it was not widely used. From the late 1930s to 1950, however, evaporated cow's milk became popular for feeding infants, among those who could afford it. In the 1950s, experimentation in the US created concentrated Similac and Enfamil formulas and provided free samples of these products to hospitals and pediatricians, which were passed on to new mothers. Although infant formula is a very deficient approximation of breast milk, mass marketing campaigns advertised it as being a modern, scientifically healthier alternative for babies. Most mothers truly believed that formula was better for their babies than breast milk. By the early 1970s, over seventy-five percent of babies in the US were fed entirely with commercially-produced formulas.[9] Infant formulas are usually made from soybeans or cow's milk (which is perfectly suited only for baby cows), and although they have been reformulated for nearly 150 years, no food substitute can come close to matching the milk made in a mother's breasts in terms of its nutrition or health-protecting qualities.

Most people now know that human breast milk is specifically created for human infants and transmits the mother's own disease immunities to protect her baby. Less well known, however, is that a mother's milk is constantly adapting to the changing needs of her baby. Breast milk automatically adjusts over time to meet all nutritional needs from those of a premature infant to those of a toddler.[10] As the baby goes through large growth spurts and needs more food, an increased volume of milk is built up in mom's breasts. If the baby is exposed to a disease, immune protection will naturally be added to the milk. In this amazingly well-coordinated interplay between mother and infant, *everything* that is needed to grow a healthy child is continuously being created within the mother's own body for the first six to twelve months of the baby's life.

Human babies typically double their birth-weight by six months and quadruple it by their third birthday. From primate studies, we know that baby monkeys are not fully weaned until they are four times heavier than at birth. Our closest ape relatives do not fully wean their infants until they weigh six times their birth weight,[11] which would be equivalent to nursing a human toddler until the child is about five years old .

Although breastfeeding is a natural act, it is also a synchronized art. In other cultures, nursing tips are passed down from mothers and grandmothers. After decades of bottle-feeding in the US, today's new mothers are at a great disadvantage. Not having built-in knowledge of breastfeeding techniques from previous generations leads many new moms to the false conclusion that they can't adequately nurse their babies. Nursing can often be difficult and painful, especially with one's first baby, as both members of the nursing couple are new to this experience. However, with educated assistance and support from other nursing moms, almost all women are able to successfully breastfeed their babies. It is important for new moms to know that licensed lactation consultants are now regularly recognized members of postpartum health teams and conveniently available throughout the US to help moms and babies become successful at nursing.

One of the most common reasons that mothers stop breastfeeding is the belief that they don't have enough milk for their babies. Just as moms are beginning to feel like they are mastering this new skill, their babies will suddenly become crankier than usual, act like they are starving, and want to eat constantly every hour around the clock. The worried mother needs to know that this is *completely normal!* Babies tend to grow in spurts and during a growth-spurt will need to consume an increased volume of milk in order to make that leap in size. While growth-spurts can occur at any time during the first year, there are typically five huge spurts: at about three weeks, six weeks, three months, six months, and nine months. When moms follow their babies' leads, their milk supplies adjust within a few days, and the babies once again become content with the new made-to-order volume of milk.

After nursing is well established, it is found to be tremendously easier, cheaper, and safer than bottle-feeding. The milk is instantly available, exactly the perfect food, always the right temperature, completely sterile, protects from illness, and very comforting to babies. A built-in advantage to a busy mother is that when nursing, she is forced to stop all other chores and just relax with her baby. Breastfeeding automatically helps one get "in tune" with her baby during these closely connected feeding times. The common term used in the US in reference to baby-initiated breastfeeding is "demand feeding." We may want to reexamine this concept because most babies elsewhere in the world don't "demand" to be nursed, but are quickly comforted at the breast whenever they desire it (see photo 9). It is common for babies throughout the world to be breastfed for at least two years and often up to five years of age. Just as babies let us know when they are ready to crawl, walk, and do other things on their own, they also let us know when they are ready to stop breastfeeding. Although my son weaned himself just after a year of age, my daughter completely regressed when I tried to wean her at age two-and-a-half. After many days of being whiny, clingy, and tearfully asking for "just a little snack," I realized she clearly was not ready to give up that source of comfort. Six months later, soon after her third birthday, she just suddenly stopped asking to nurse any more.

The World Health Organization (WHO) and the American Academy of Pediatrics (AAP) recommend exclusive breastfeeding for the first *six months* of an infant's life to achieve the best growth, development, and overall health. Feeding the baby *only breast milk,* and no other liquids, formula, or solid foods for six months has strong advantages over only three to four months of exclusive breastfeeding or mixing breastfeeding with formula or any solid foods.[12] In 2011 the WHO stated that a baby who is exclusively breastfed without the introduction of *any* formula for at least the first six months, has a much lower risk of gastrointestinal infections. After the introduction of solid foods at six months, continuing to breastfeed is recommended by both the WHO and AAP until the child is at least two years old. "Breastfeeding is an unequalled way of providing ideal food for the healthy growth and development of infants . . . Malnutrition throughout the world has been responsible, directly or indirectly, for sixty percent of the 10.9 million deaths annually of children under five. Well over two-thirds of these deaths, which are often associated with inappropriate feeding practices, occur during the first year of life."[13]

Robin Lim, an American midwife and 2011 CNN Hero of the Year for her work creating birthing clinics in communities challenged by natural and man-made disasters, has lived in Bali for over twenty years. On my 2004 trip to Bali I spent an afternoon with "Ibu (Mother) Robin" at her Balinese birthing clinic. One of Robin's greatest concerns was that even in Bali, babies were beginning to become malnourished due to the recently introduced practice of using formula to feed babies after the terrorist bombing disrupted the economy. It is terribly immoral for Western companies take advantage of peoples' suffering by introducing products that can cause harm. A Balinese baby fed infant formula is three hundred times more likely to die in the first year of life as compared to a breastfed infant.[14]

Sudden Infant Death Syndrome (SIDS) is the unexpected death of a child under one year of age in which an autopsy does not show an explainable cause. A recent study of SIDS in Germany found that breastfeeding reduced the risk of SIDS by approximately fifty percent throughout infancy and recommended that "SIDS risk-reduction messages" always be included in advice about the importance of breastfeeding through at least six months of age.[15] In 2012, the AAP passed a resolution advising

American pediatricians not to provide formula samples or coupons to the parents of infants. The AAP states that patients must be protected from commercial infant formula marketing since research has found that such gifts adversely affect breastfeeding exclusivity and duration.[16]

The natural spacing between children, aided by two to five years of breastfeeding, which usually inhibits ovulation, ensures that babies get the time and attention they need before having to compete with a new sibling. Unfortunately for dads, this is also helped by the fact that the hormones promoted while breastfeeding usually cause moms to have a nonexistent sex-drive. The previous generation's popular two-year spacing of children in Western cultures coincided with the usage of formula so sex-drive and ovulation wasn't affected. As a psychologist, I recommend at least a four-year spacing between children, since being able to meet a toddler's needs greatly reduces sibling rivalry. Siblings one and a half to three and a half years apart tend to have the most intense problems with rivalry. An attachment can definitely be stressed by the birth of another baby too soon. Tired parents usually expect toddlers to act much older than they can, but two-year-olds can't even share a cookie, let alone a mother!

Fathers can have a huge influence on whether their babies are breast-fed. It is important that Western fathers understand, as those in the peaceful cultures do, that in addition to the physical benefits, his baby is also receiving social and emotional advantages when suckling from his mother. Breastfeeding is the most intimate form of skin-to-skin contact, and so provides a high dose of the love hormones oxytocin and prolactin in a nursing mother, which stimulate calm, nurturing, and protective feelings toward her infant. Since the breastfeeding baby also receives these hormones, a close suckling relationship promotes feelings of contentment, safety, and trust within the baby. When new mothers must return to work and diligently pump breast milk during each break to later be bottle-fed to their baby, these skin-to-skin based benefits are missing. Policy makers need to understand that new moms and babies would benefit much more from paid maternity leaves rather than all the time and money that has gone into developing fancier, more efficient breast pumps. Research indicates that when fathers are supportive of their

## Health Benefits of Breastfeeding

**For moms** who exclusively breastfeed for the first 6 months:[17]

- Decreases in postpartum bleeding
- Easier loss of pregnancy weight
- A reduction in the probability of ovulation (protecting a new mom from getting pregnant again until she has fully recovered)

Breastfeeding is associated with a reduction in the mother's future risk of:[18]

- Ovarian and breast cancer
- Anemia
- Osteoporosis
- Type II diabetes

Not breastfeeding or stopping early is correlated with an increased risk of:[19]

- Maternal postpartum depression

**For babies** it is associated with **a reduction in:**[20]

- Childhood cancers including leukemia
- Necrotizing enterocolitis (bowel tissue death seen primarily in premature infants)
- Non-specific gastroenteritis (acute diarrhea and vomiting.)
- Severe lower respiratory tract infections
- Childhood asthma
- Obesity
- Type I and II diabetes
- Ear infections
- Atopic dermatitis (a type of eczema)
- SIDS

babies being breastfed, even when mothers return to work outside of the home, over ninety-eight percent of mothers will continue breastfeeding their infants and toddlers. But if the dads are indifferent to breastfeeding, only 26.9 percent of moms continue to nurse their babies.[21] In the first few weeks of learning how to breastfeed, exhausted new mothers often question whether they can successfully nurse their babies. Having partners who are encouraging, and remind them that it will get easier once babies are bit older and won't be nursing so often, can really make a big difference in terms of moms forging onward.

Close maternal attachment is correlated with prolonged breastfeeding providing the baby with optimal advantages in physical and emotional health. In all of the world's peaceful cultures, breastfeeding is regarded as time during which the mother is feeding love to her baby. The Dalai Lama believes, "From the very day of our births, when we drink our mother's milk, compassion arises within us. This act is a symbol of love and affection. I think this act, from the very first day of life, establishes the basis for all other relationships throughout our entire life."[22]

## Wearing Babies

A baby wants to be in close bodily contact with his mother, father, or primary caregiver. For the first nine months of his life, a human infant is a lot like a baby kangaroo, which is born much too soon to fend for itself and lives in a pouch attached to its mom's body which simulates still being in the womb. Being born in a similar premature state, human infants have a deep need for the type of carrying and movement that is similar to being in the womb. Tibetans and Balinese believe that continuous bodily contact with one's mother, father, and other members of the family are essential for healthy mental and emotional development. Babies crave constant physical and emotional connections and feel most secure when they are "worn" on their parents' bodies. In the US, new parents spend a lot of money on baby furniture—infant seats, bouncy chairs, swings, and fancy strollers—but all an infant usually wants is to be worn in a simple sling.

Babies in most of the world are carried in slings on the front or side of a parent's body for the first year, and carried on a parent's back for the next few years (see photo 10). This close contact makes it easy for parents to talk with and soothe the baby. When babies are "worn," they tend to cry less and are more easily comforted. Parenting is clearly more stressful when babies are fretful or screaming, so anything that comforts a baby is also comforting to the parents. Content babies are just simply easier for everyone to enjoy, thus baby-wearing promotes more positive parent-infant connections.

## Co-Sleeping

The practice of sleeping with or nearby your infant, while still controversial and long resisted in the US, is for most people in the world a naturally accepted practice. Tibetan children spend most of the day with a loving family member and sleep in the same bed as their parents until they are about seven years old. Naho told me that in Japan, infants tend to sleep in a crib right next to their parents' sleeping futon until they are old enough to climb out, and then they sleep between their parents on the futon. She said that it is common for parents to lie down with infants and young children until they fall asleep.[23] In Bali, Nyoman spoke of how babies and toddlers always sleep in bed with their parents. When children are older, they sleep on special floor mats in the family sleeping room until they are teenagers. When we spoke, Nyoman was feeling sad because her son, at age fourteen, had just asked to leave the family sleeping room and have a room of his own in the family compound. It is in this new room that his wife and children will sleep when he later becomes married. The Balinese love the closeness of a family sharing a sleeping room, which seems much like how Western families feel when they go camping and sleep together in a tent.[24] In Bhutan, children sleep in a large bed with their parents until they are between four and seven years of age. Children's cries are always gently responded to during the daytime or nighttime. Dr. Mimi told me that she had been sorry to hear that American babies are only allowed to sleep in the same bed as their parents during their first year. She was clearly shocked when I told her that actually, most American parents never sleep with their children.[25]

The US consistently stands out as the only society in which babies at even a few months of age are often placed in their own beds and in their own rooms.[26] Americans are confused by the term "co-sleeping," wondering what exactly it means. I identify co-sleeping as having two components: "room-sharing" and "bed-sharing." "Room-sharing" means having the baby sleep in the same room within arm's reach of a parent, while "bed-sharing" means the baby sleeps in the same bed as the parents. While room-sharing is becoming more of an accepted practice by Western parents, most room-sharers also at times become bed-sharers. It is very difficult for tired parents not to fall asleep with their babies, even if they are not intending to do so. The historical controversy in the US concerning bed-sharing, leaves some well-meaning parents fearful of sleeping with their babies and if they do so, they often feel guilty and try to hide it from others.

The largest study conducted to-date on Sudden Infant Death Syndrome (SIDS) found that the risk of death for infants who slept in their parents' bedroom was about half that of infants who slept alone.[27] Recent studies from Great Britain, New Zealand, and a number of other Western European countries concur that babies who do not room-share, but are left in a crib in their own room without supervision for long periods of time, are nearly *twice as likely* to die of SIDS.[28] In fact, "most cultures that routinely practice co-sleeping in any form have very rare instances of SIDS."[29] Some room-sharing parents put their babies in a bassinet next to the bed, a "co-sleeper" that opens to the side of the adult bed, or in a basket that is set in bed between the two parents. Extensive and rigorous scientific studies have determined that room-sharing is not only normal and instinctive, but may be the very best way for a family to protect and nurture infants, because if an infant experiences any distress, the parents will instantly be aware that there is a problem. Most cultures combine room-sharing with bed-sharing, and in actuality, bed-sharing has many benefits and little risk if safety measures are followed.

It is natural throughout the world for a mother to bed-share with her baby to observe that the baby is safe, and even to breastfeed intermittently throughout the night. Breastfeeding is much easier if a baby is sleeping next her mother's body, and helps mom's sleep be less interrupted. One of the greatest causes of postpartum depression and anxiety in new moms is from not getting enough sleep. Adequate rest is vital to a new mother's mood, and helps increase positive feelings rather than resentment toward her newborn. When done safely, mother-infant bed-sharing with nightly breastfeeding nicely meets both the infant's and the mother's needs.

Nighttime contact promotes feelings of connection between parents and their youngsters, which goes a long way in building emotional equity for those times when things get difficult. Just as adults typically enjoy sleeping next to someone, infants and young children have an even stronger need and desire for this type of closeness during the night. If a youngster is going through a stressful time or spending many hours each day away from her parents, being kept close during the night can be especially reassuring and help them reconnect. All mammals sleep with their young; in fact, we would consider them neglectful if they didn't. Imagine a mother cat leaving her whimpering kittens alone while she slept in another room. Wouldn't we feel sorry for those kittens and be worried about their survival? If a mother cat can sleep safely with her kittens, shouldn't we assume that most mother humans could do the same?

For the past twenty years, research on the differences between solitary and co-sleeping mother-infant pairs have been conducted with funding from the National Institute of Child Health and Human Development. Of special interest has been how sleeping arrangements affect mothers' and infants' nighttime physiology and behavior.[30] Dr. James McKenna, an anthropologist and the director of the University of Notre Dame's Mother-Baby Behavioral Sleep Laboratory, has found that, since human infants are born incredibly underdeveloped compared to other mammals, they are neither "biologically designed nor prepared to be separated from their mothers," especially while sleeping.[31] McKenna explains that in Asian, African, Central and South American, and southern European countries, bed-sharing is the norm until children are weaned and often for much longer. Dr. McKenna wants "families to understand how much happens during sleep and bed-sharing, including contact with each other through touch, scent, sound, and taste. This unconscious communication is part of the way our species has evolved to maximize health and survival. A baby sleeping alone in a crib outside the supervision and monitoring of its mother or father is deprived of this vital communication and is, therefore, as scientific studies have shown, at increased risk."[32]

A baby with an immature respiratory system will definitely benefit from sleeping near his mother because the sound and chest movements of the mother's breathing can assist the baby to develop steady rhythmic breathing. Remember, babies are just learning how to breathe and some of them need extra help. Even the carbon dioxide that a mother exhales helps stimulate her baby's breathing, as long as the mother has not been smoking cigarettes.

When in the same bed, being breastfed every few hours, an infant is inclined to spend less time in deep sleep states that can be risky until breathing has been mastered. Babies that sleep near their mothers spend more time in lighter states of sleep, which are believed to be safer for young infants. When babies are kept in close proximity to their parents, any difficulties in respiration can be more readily detected and interventions quickly made. Numerous studies have shown that "when resting on their mothers' torsos, both premature and full-term infants breathe more regularly, use energy more efficiently, maintain lower blood pressure, grow faster, and experience less stress."[33]

Since 2005, the American Academy of Pediatrics (AAP) has recommended room-sharing as a way to reduce SIDS. While research points to the increase in safety of having infants room-share with their parents for at least the first six months of life, this does not mean all families should bed-share. Dr. McKenna stresses the importance of educating families as to safe co-sleeping practices and *to avoid bed-sharing* when adverse conditions pose risks for the infant.[34] While a mother usually responds if her baby moves into a dangerous position, is making unusual noises or stops breathing, it is critical that she and any adult sharing the bed adhere to each of the following safety factors.

## Assure that Your Baby is as Safe as Possible[37, 38]

- Always lay the baby on her back, the natural and safest position for breastfeeding and sleeping.
- Make sure that no one smokes in your home, around the baby, or holds the baby even after smoking outside. (Secondhand smoke is in the air, and third-hand smoke is on hands, clothing, or one's breath—

and *all* are dangerous for a baby.) Exhalations by a smoker during sleep can hinder a baby's breathing. If the mother smoked during her pregnancy or if either parent currently smokes, they should avoid bed-sharing.

- Use a firm mattress with tight-fitting sheets.
- Keep pillows, soft blankets, bumper pads, and stuffed animals away from baby's face.
- Do not put the baby to sleep on soft surfaces such as a couch, recliner, waterbed, pillow, or beanbag chair.
- Make sure there is no space between the bed and wall where the baby could roll and become trapped.
- Consider placing a firm mattress on the floor in the middle of the room to prevent the baby from falling off or becoming trapped between mattress and wall or headboard.
- Do not let the baby get overheated from too warm a room or being overly bundled. (Overheating is associated with an increased risk of SIDS.)
- Do not bed-share with other children or pets while the baby is less than one year old.
- Always keep the baby close enough to see or hear him if problems arise.
- Share this information with everyone who cares for your baby and may lay down with her to sleep

## *Never* Bed-Share with Your Baby if You (or any bed-sharing adult): [39, 40]

- Smoke.
- Have consumed alcohol or other drugs that may alter consciousness.
- Take sedatives or medications that cause drowsiness.
- Are very tired or ill and may not wake up easily.
- Are markedly obese. (There is increased risk of obese parents accidently lying on their babies, because they may not be able to feel how close they are to the baby.)

For parents with any of these risk factors, the use of "co-sleepers," which are crib-like beds that are the same height and can sit next to and open to the parents' bed would provide a much safer alternative. Of concern for many bed-sharing parents is whether they will ever be able to get their child out of their bed. All children at some point inherently want independence from their parents. We know that even babies who are held a lot will, at some point, squirm their way out of arms and demand to be put down so they can crawl, walk, and run. The same is true for co-sleeping children; they all will at some point want their own bed in their own room. One study, however, found that the acceptance of solitary sleeping by co-sleeping children came about a year later than for children who were solitary sleepers from birth. In exchange for one year longer of co-sleeping, you can help your child become more self-sufficient, resilient, secure, and have a greater comfort with affectional touch.[41]

One problem many new parents wonder about is how they can ever be sexually intimate when they're room-sharing, especially if bed-sharing, with their child. Well, in most of the co-sleeping cultures I have visited, the bedroom is *not* considered the place for sexual intimacy. It is more like a family room, not a place for nighttime parental intimacy as it is viewed in Western countries. The sleeping room is a place of affection, touching, hugging, cuddling, and feeling close for all family members. It appears that couples in co-sleeping cultures creatively find other places to have exciting erotic rendezvous.

## Affection

All humans crave affection. When we receive positive touch, gentle words, hugs, kisses, and cuddles, love hormones released into our bodies create contentment, warmth, and an overall sense of well-being. For crying babies, receiving affection, kindness, and knowing they are being listened to, usually calms them, just like it does for people of any age. Besides providing comfort, touching and gently stroking babies has the additional benefit of building brain connections that increase the children's ability to calm themselves when older.[42]

The Tibetans have long known that touch is extremely important to a baby for bonding and brain development. Bhutanese infants and toddlers are given constant attention and affection. When they're not in their parents' arms, the babies are usually being carried around by their older siblings (see photo 11).[43] Parenting in extended families helps babies receive lots of love from others, thereby leaving the mother less stressed and more able to be nurturing when the baby is with her.

Affection is so important to the Balinese that an infant is constantly held in someone's arms for the first three months of life, and I have rarely seen a child in Bali under three years of age not being carried by someone (see photo 12). In Bali it is an honor to hold a baby. I realized that I had gained a new level of acceptance by my "Balinese family" on my last visit there, when babies were being given to me for holding. I felt very honored when the family's tiny twelve-day-old infant was handed to me immediately upon my arrival. At another baby's forty-two-day naming ceremony, I was pronounced a "pintar Ibu" (clever mother) when the newly named baby boy was relaxed and content in my arms. After his ceremony, I delightfully sat on the veranda celebrating with the villagers as the little baby slept in my arms for over an hour and a half. Surrounded by happy families with their joyful children's clear eyes and open-hearted spirits warmed my heart. I remember feeling that this gentle parenting and cherishing of babies was without a doubt creating delightfully kind kids.

Affection helps babies learn to give and receive love. Isn't it obvious which of our acquaintances were treated affectionately as children? Children treated with tenderness develop the ability to be compassionate and empathetic, a gift in all their future relationships.[44] Trust me, when you treat your children with affection, their future friends, spouses, and children will be extremely grateful to you!

## Listening and Responding

Newborns are so completely dependent on their caregivers that they can't even scratch an itch during the first few months of life. Due to their extreme immaturity at birth, our babies are not at all able to regulate their internal emotions, so the idea that infants can be taught to "self calm" if left unattended is simply incorrect. When a newborn cries, he is trying to communicate his need for parental assistance to be fed, held, warmed, comforted, changed, burped, etc. If babies are comforted whenever they get stressed, they will eventually learn smooth patterns of regulation. If when hungry they get fed, if when cold they are warmed, if when tired they are rocked to sleep, neural connections in their brains begin developing that will help them be able to self-calm in emotional, behavioral, or mental situations when they are older.[45] There are those who caution parents not pick up a baby "just because it wants attention." But, even if a baby does *just* want attention, why is that bad? Wanting attention is a basic condition of being a social animal. Don't we all just want and need attention sometimes? Imagine if you'd had a hard day and asked your husband for a hug, and he responded, "I'm not going to hug you just because you want attention!" That probably wouldn't go a long way in creating comfort or trust in your relationship.

While a parent can't always respond immediately every time a baby cries, it is important for the parent to reassure the baby that you hear her and are coming to help as soon as you can. Listening and responding teaches a baby that her needs are important. In the first eighteen months of life, an infant is learning whether she can trust others to "be there" when she needs them. Knowing that those who care about you will try to help creates feelings of self-worth along with trust in relationships. Babies who develop this type of trust begin their lives believing they are worthy and that relationships are comforting, safe, and dependable.[46]

Some parenting programs encourage the use of "controlled crying techniques" as an attempt to teach babies to calm down and get themselves to sleep. The "Cry It Out" (CIO) approach was first suggested in 1895.[47] CIO often refers to any sleep-training method in which a baby is either not responded to at all or allowed to cry for a specified time before receiving any comfort from a caregiver. While babies will eventually cry themselves to sleep, they are simultaneously learning that their caregivers are not trustworthy. This is extremely confusing and frightening for a baby. Many of today's child development specialists believe that any method using CIO is unnatural, unnecessary, and may create potentially serious problems.[48] Responding to crying babies is so natural to parents in peaceful cultures that even the concept of allowing a baby to "cry it out" would be unimaginable. The Australian Association for Infant Mental Health has issued a warning that controlled crying is not consistent with what infants need for optimal emotional and psychological health, and suggests that it may have unintended negative consequences.[49] Prolonged crying dramatically increases cortisol, an adrenal hormone related to stress. Some studies have suggested that elevated cortisol in an infant's brain may cause detachment leading to later problems in socialization and relationships.[50]

## Singing and Playing

Singing, playing, and talking with your baby is essential for healthy brain development. The best time to talk and play with a newborn is when they are in a "quiet alert state" of consciousness. Watch for this state of alertness when your infant is calm, quiet, not moving his body, and has his eyes wide open looking around. Even a newborn can recognize your voice and face, turning toward you for eye contact. In this state he is very aware, open to observing, and will turn toward your voice, gaze into your eyes, and may even imitate your facial expression. Eyes are particularly fascinating to a newborn and they love to gaze into yours. A newborn's ability to see is much better than was once believed, especially at a distance of about twelve inches, probably not coincidently, the distance from mom's breast to her eyes. Engaging your baby in these short periods of focused visual attention is your first direct communication with him. These moments are extremely enjoyable, exciting, and mark the beginning of your intimate relationship.[51]

Music and play are used in every world culture to create closeness, change moods, and lift spirits. The ancient practice of soothing babies through song has led to the great number of lullabies created for just that purpose. Music and rhythms organize basic brain structures in babies that later help toddlers in being able to think and speak. Babies love to be sung to, but don't worry if you can't carry a tune—they are not music critics!

Karta, an incredible artist in Bali, a culture known to have some of the most creative people on the planet, believes that we must try to remember what it feels like to be a child in order to recall what children need. He states that at least until age five, 90 percent of a child's time should be spent playing. His wise words are cautionary, "Keeping children laughing, playing, and happy helps their brains grow. But TV, computers, and video games make the brain lazy, they keep it from growing creative."[52] It is delightful to watch how the Balinese adults love running around playing and teasing the children. I often noticed that although the Balinese love to dress up in their most beautiful native clothes for their many ceremonies, the young children are usually not dressed in fancy clothes. When I questioned this at a family wedding, my Balinese "son" Narok explained, "When children are little they like to play, and that's what is most important. It is much easier to play when not dressed-up. Kids start wearing elegant Balinese clothes after they finish elementary school."[53]

When parents comfort babies with song, dance, and play, they create closer attachments and babies delight in spending time with them. Likewise, a baby who responds, smiles, and is thrilled to see his parent triggers an increased desire to spend even more time with that baby. Relationships are reciprocal, and we all crave positive loving connections. Caregivers who spend lots of time playing with their babies (peekaboo, this little piggy, the bee is getting the tummy, etc.) help them become delightful children who are playful, joyful, and fun to be around. Such personality types benefit by having more positive social relationships, and happier, more optimistic lives.

## Close Proximity

Babies need to be kept in close proximity to their caregivers, particularly the first nine months after birth, while they are completely at the mercy of their caregivers for their basic survival. Other mammals stay close to their newborns during this vulnerable early stage of life and are extremely protective of them. Monkey babies are usually riding on their mother's body, as do human babies in cultures where they are customarily worn in a sling. From my observations and those of others, at one month of age the amount of time a baby spends alone is zero for a Balinese, 8.3 percent for a Korean, and 67.5 percent for an American.[54]

It became a common practice in the US during previous generations (and is still suggested by some pediatricians) to put a baby in its *own* room at a few months of age and not to respond when the baby cries during the night. Most mothers around the world keep their babies in sight and hearing at all times day and night in order to help immediately if any need or problem arises. The idea of putting a baby in another room to sleep or "self-calm" would be considered neglect in most of the world. Could this American practice of not responding to a crying baby during the night be related to our high infant mortality rate? I recently heard about a baby who had died of SIDS after the well-meaning mother had put the baby to bed in his own room and did not check on him for over ten hours. The infant mortality rate in the US is considerably greater than other countries in the world, with forty-five other developed countries having a lower rate than ours.[55] SIDS is one of three leading causes of infant death in the US (in 2010 there were more than two thousand unexplained infant deaths).[56]

In light of these facts, it seems that one of the easiest preventive measures would be to keep your infant nearby at all times during his first, and most vulnerable, year of life. If a baby is just lightly fussing, he may be able to get himself back to sleep, but if he starts crying loudly, he clearly needs help. Similarly, if a baby chokes or stops breathing, it is critically important that someone be nearby to recognize and respond to this emergency.

In most of the world, sleeping babies are never put in another room or placed out of range from eyes and ears of a caregiving family member. Even in Nepal, one of the poorest countries in the world, where mothers are working so hard that they often can't be directly caring for their babies, someone is usually watching out for them. High in a Himalayan village, I observed one-year-old Ganji being carried on her older sister's back while the teen worked as a server in the family restaurant (see photo 13). When this sister was at school and her mom was in the kitchen cooking, Ganji spent time in a small crib placed in the middle of the restaurant dining area so that everyone, including the guests, could interact with her.

In addition to avoiding potential dangers that could occur due to your not having your baby close-by, your baby will thrive physically and emotionally when kept in close proximity to you. Keeping your baby close throughout the day and night will encourage more interaction, talking, playing, and responding to each other. This type of intimacy not only leads to increased social awareness and the earlier development of language skills, but also naturally encourages a strong, secure, and positive attachment.

## Factors that Inhibit Attachment

Along with knowing what promotes attachments between new parents and their offspring, it seems important to also understand what interferes with it. A woman who has just given birth has experienced one of the most strenuous, exhausting, and painful challenges that is humanly possible. This new mother likely feels both infinitely powerful and exceedingly vulnerable. If the birth went as planned, she can experience the success of a physically demanding undertaking comparable to climbing the highest mountain in the world. She is also being initiated into the awe-inspiring but equally mystifying and sometimes terrifying life-stage of motherhood. Will she be able to meet all the needs of this tiny new being and help him grow into a healthy, capable, loving, moral, and contributing member of society? The hormones surging through her body open her heart wide, ready to love her newborn miracle, but she also feels extremely exposed and sensitive to everything that is happening around her.

---

### Factors That Inhibit Attachment

- Unplanned Pregnancy
- Difficult Birth
- Lack of Hormonal Support
- Low Apgar Score
- Baby Different from Imagined
- Hospital Routines
- Negative Comments
- Parents' Own Attachments
- Postpartum Mood Disorder
- Fear of Spoiling

---

Some factors that can inhibit attachment often occur at the very beginning of a parent-baby relationship and may include: an unplanned pregnancy, an unusually difficult birth, lack of hormonal support, a low newborn Apgar score, when a baby is very different from the one imagined, intrusive hospital routines, negative comments from the hospital staff or visitors, a parent's insecure attachments to his or her own parents, postpartum depression or anxiety, and a socially-imposed fear of spoiling the child. It seems important to describe the potential impact of these influences, because most new parents have great angst when they don't feel a close heart-to-heart connection with their newborn, and don't realize that these commonly occurring factors may have hindered the natural attachment process. If anything has interfered, parents can still promote a strong attachment by beginning to implement as many as possible of the Global Practices that Increase Attachments listed in the previous section of this chapter.

## Unplanned Pregnancy

The Balinese and Bhutanese encourage the use of birth control for family planning and the Tibetans have a special focus on preconception preparation of body and mind along with expectations that conception should occur during a gentle, loving union in which a baby's spirit is invited to enter. In the US, however, forty-nine percent of pregnancies are unintended, with twenty-nine percent of these being mistimed, and nineteen percent being entirely unwanted.[57] When a woman finds out that she is pregnant without planning this major life-changing event, she can feel very confused, overwhelmed, anxious, fearful, and depressed. Perhaps she believed, up to this point in life, that she had complete control of her life choices and decisions. She is suddenly faced with one of the most significant life-altering experiences, which she did not choose, at least not at that moment in time. Is she ready to be a mother? Can she successfully be the mother this baby needs? Does she have financial and emotional support? A woman in this situation sometimes faces abandonment by the baby's father and/or by her own family and friends. The young woman often begins such a pregnancy feeling isolated and alone. If she decides to continue with the pregnancy, she may harbor doubt and even resentment toward the baby.

Prenatal depression and anxiety are very common throughout unintended pregnancies. A pregnant woman is often afraid to even let others know about her fears and negative feelings, convincing herself that they serve as proof that she will be an inadequate mother. This new mom is also at high risk for developing a depressive or anxious mood disorder after the birth and may find difficulty attaching to her newborn. Seeking counseling and/or social support during and after the pregnancy can help a mother in this situation be more accepting of her baby.

## Difficult Birth

One's birthing experience is definitely an important initiation to mothering. If a woman feels that she has some control of the birth process, with her own feelings and requests being honored, birthing a baby can be an incredibly empowering experience. A successful birthing experience can leave a woman strongly confident that she can handle anything, which is necessary, because mothers *do* need to be able to handle everything! A difficult birth that ends up with interventions that the mother did not want might leave her feeling inadequate or that her body has failed her and the baby. Such feelings can interfere with a new mom's ability to attach to her infant.

There are two models of birthing care in the United States. Midwives are specialists in assisting with low-risk pregnancy, childbirth, and postpartum care. They encourage good nutrition, healthy exercise, and reduced stress, and do their best to reduce fears of childbirth that often accompany beliefs that human women's bodies are not able to birth their young as well as other mammals can. Midwives spend much time with a woman getting to know her, understand her fears, and educate her about bodily changes, fetal development, and the body's well-designed ability to give birth, and to assist her in developing feelings of attachment to her unborn baby. Traditionally, midwives try to keep women well-informed and supported throughout their pregnancies, birth experiences, and postpartum care. A certified nurse midwife has a master of science degree in nursing with specialized training as a primary healthcare provider for healthy women whose births are not considered "high risk." Midwives are trained to recognize abnormal complications of pregnancy and will refer women to an obstetrician if they require care beyond the midwife's scope of expertise.

An obstetrician, on the other hand, is a surgeon who has excellent training in dealing with possible complications related to childbearing. Ideally, these two professions could serve very complementary roles in women's pregnancies. All too often, however, there is not only a lack of cooperation but even animosity due to fundamental differences in their approaches to birth and the fact that the US was the only country in the world that ever tried to eliminate midwifery. While midwives are trained to allow births to proceed naturally and will not intervene unless necessary, obstetricians are taught to actively manage births. An obstetrician-managed birth typically involves medical interventions, currently including the use of Pitocin, a synthetic hormone administered intravenously to speed up and control uterine contractions, and an epidural, a spinal analgesia administered to alleviate pain. Birth interventions can increase the risk of complications and lead to an emergency cesarean (C-section) birth.

A recent study released by the National Institute of Child Health and Human Development found that C-section rates become *twice as high* after an induction of labor as compared with labor that is allowed to begin naturally.[58] A cesarean involves major abdominal surgery, definitely a life-saving technique for the mother and/or baby if a serious medical emergency arises, but should never be chosen under the mistaken belief that they are "easier and safer" than vaginal births or "better for the baby." A woman deserves to be informed that a C-section involves weeks of painful healing and carries the potential for serious medical complications. While most C-sections proceed without difficulty, increased risks to the mother's health include possible problems with anesthesia, infection, hemorrhage, need for blood transfusions, injury to other internal organs, fatal pulmonary embolisms, and psychological difficulties. A vaginal birth has always been the safest way for a baby to be born. Maternal mortality is three times higher for elective and four times higher for emergency cesarean births. The World Health Organization (WHO) states that no region in the world should have a cesarean rate greater than ten to fifteen percent,[59] however, the C-section rate in the US is currently close to thirty-four percent, with births attended by midwives having a cesarean rate of less than five percent. This means that a pregnant mother with an obstetrician-managed birth has a one in three chance of having a C-section as compared to a one in twenty chance with a midwife.

Scotland, the Netherlands, and Scandinavian countries have continued to keep their C-section and maternal death rates some of the lowest in the world.[60] In Bali, midwife Robin Lim's birthing clinic, Bumi Sehat (Heavenly Earth Mother), provides extensive support to promote healthy birth outcomes. Pregnant mothers are offered prenatal checkups, supportive and caring birth experiences, postpartum care, and breastfeeding support, all free of charge. The birthing clinic was created to reduce maternal and infant mortality rates, and provide much more positive birth experiences than women were receiving in the hospital.[61]

In the past decade, a much higher percentage of "elective" births began being induced by American obstetricians several weeks prior to a baby's actual due date. These inductions were often arranged for convenience due to the doctor or pregnant mother's schedule and sometimes merely because the mother was tired of being pregnant (commonly termed "TOP Syndrome," meaning "Tired Of Pregnancy"). While I have never met a woman who isn't tired of being pregnant by the end of the third trimester, shortening a pregnancy increases risks to the baby in terms of weight, vision, development of lungs and brain, and interference with natural initiation of breastfeeding, which can then lead to dehydration and jaundice. Babies born before term, whether as result of prematurity, early induction, or elective cesarean are more likely to need breathing-machine assistance after the birth and are nearly twice as likely to spend time in a neonatal intensive care unit (NICU).[62] Human mothers, just like other mammal mothers, who are deprived of immediate contact with their newborns because of procedures that result in the baby being removed, often have difficulty attaching to them later. Early separation due to infant distress which results in disrupting a mother's feelings of connection can remain disturbed during the first year or more of the infant's life, even when the baby's health problems are completely resolved within a few hours.[63]

Chapters of the American Congress of Obstetricians and Gynecologists in 2010 alerted doctors as to the serious consequences for babies born from early elective births. In California, collaboration between the Department of Public Health, the Maternal Quality Care Collaborative, and the March of Dimes, has called for the elimination of all elective deliveries or C-sections prior to thirty-nine weeks of gestation.[64]

Medical intervention during childbirth can also lead to other psychological difficulties with normal bonding and attachment, because these more easily occur when a new mother feels positive about her birth experience. Pride in the way she was able to move through this important rite-of-passage, along with the cascade of naturally occurring hormones released during a non-medicated birth, creates the most favorable circumstances for a mother to experience an immediate love-bond with her baby. Rest assured, however, if you don't feel an immediate attachment, by realizing that the newborn has also gone through an especially difficult transition, and that by trying to gently reassure and respond to the baby, the relationship between you can become a mutually healing and loving one.

## Lack of Hormonal Support

A woman's body automatically releases a mixture of hormones during an undisturbed labor and delivery that assists the mother emotionally throughout the birth by helping her to both cope with the pain and also feel a close connection to her baby. When a woman feels safe and supported, and receives loving, kind understanding, she is able to enter a relaxed trance-like state that allows for the optimal release of a hormonal birthing cocktail that assists her throughout the birth. Midwives and doulas are extremely useful in helping a birthing mother to enter into this state.

The four major birthing hormones are endorphins, oxytocin, adrenaline, noradrenaline, and prolactin. Beta-endorphin is nature's opiate that provides natural pain relief and an altered state of consciousness along with promoting feelings of pleasure and connectedness. Oxytocin, which gradually increases during labor and reaches a peak at the birth, causes uterine contractions and stimulates feelings of love in the mother toward her infant. Adrenaline and noradrenaline assist with the stressful physical demands while protecting the baby during powerful contractions. Prolactin offers gentle nurturing feelings that peak for both the mother and baby at birth and when the baby begins to suckle at the mother's breast. Our hormonal systems that are activated during labor and delivery enhance the birthing experience, safely guide its progression, and help the mother and baby to experience a heart-opening natural attachment.[65]

When Pitocin (a synthetic oxytocin) is injected in a laboring mother to increase uterine contractions, an epidural is administered for pain relief, or other interventions are used to manage labor, interference with the naturally occurring hormones often leave the mother and baby at a grave disadvantage. Pitocin, which is used to induce or speed up labor, makes contractions longer, stronger, and closer together than would naturally occur, resulting in greater pain. The medications then given for pain relief hinder the beta-endorphin release, which would have naturally provided comfort and positive feelings of goodwill. If a mother becomes fearful, the brain receives signals that there is danger and, attempting to protect the birthing pair, the labor will automatically slow down or even stop.[66] All of these conditions can keep the baby from getting sufficient oxygen, thus leading to fetal distress and precipitating the need for an emergency caesarean.

When a laboring mother's normal hormonal physiology is disturbed by externally supplied medications, it interferes with the naturally occurring hormonal cocktail that has been finely tuned over millions of years to support her during the birthing process. This lack of normal hormonal support can alter the birth, leaving a new mom feeling emotionally depleted, detached, and sometimes even resentful of her newborn. One such disempowered mother of a medically-induced birth that resulted in many complications, sadly asked me, "How was I supposed to love that baby who had just caused me to suffer more than I have ever suffered in my life?" She had been deprived of her body's own natural hormonal support that could have led to feelings of empowerment, ecstasy, and love. Instead, she was left feeling angry, resentful, and detached from her newborn.

## Low Apgar Score or Baby Different from Imagined

An attending doctor or midwife gives each newborn an "Apgar score" in the first minute after the birth and again at five minutes. This score is based on an observation of the baby's *Appearance*, *Pulse*, *Grimace*, *Activity*, and *Respiration*, each factor being scored from zero to two points. Scores of seven to ten are considered normal, four to six are fairly low, with three and below being critically concerning. When these scores are low, a parent's feelings of attachment will often be delayed due to fears that something is seriously wrong with the baby.

Parental attachment to babies often begins during the pregnancies. Early attached parents usually have strong impressions of what their baby is like. If, after being born, a newborn appears very different from what was imagined (by gender, looks, or any birth abnormalities), attachment can be affected. Parents often need time to make the shift from the imagined baby to the actual baby before they are able to comfortably attach to their infant. Delayed attachment can take days, weeks, or even months, so new parents should be patient if they don't immediately feel in love their baby.

## Hospital Routines

Hospitals often have a number of procedures that are routinely followed within a certain period before and after a birth, which can be disruptive to attachment. Expectant parents can alter some of these routines by presenting their doctor or midwife with a written birth plan delineating exactly what they do and do not want done during their infant's birthing experience. Knowing, for instance, that the first ninety minutes after birth, while the baby is in the "quiet alert state," is a critical time for attachment, parents, doulas, and birth attendants can strongly advocate that bathing, weighing, phenylketonuria (PKU) testing to determine if the baby has an enzyme needed for normal development, and other intrusive routines be delayed until after the newborn has been welcomed during this brief but important stage. The first hour after the birth is a very special time when the parents and baby are falling in love with each other. It is important for them to have uninterrupted privacy during these precious moments to begin their relationship as a family.

## Negative Comments

When a mom has just given birth and oxytocin is priming her to fall in love with her baby, she is especially open and trusting of everyone around her. Those in attendance should be careful of the comments they make at such a vulnerable time, because they can have a powerful influence on a mother's feelings toward her baby. Observations made by others can affect the new mom at a deep subconscious level. (Remember when you were first falling in love and how sensitive you were to any comments made about that person.) If someone remarks that a new son seems "very determined," it could be much more helpful to the mom's attachment than a comment about him being "really demanding." In the following weeks, when that exhausted mom is awakened by her son's cries four times a night, the words spoken at his birth may play loudly in her mind and can affect her feelings toward him.

A mother once told me that she was haunted for years after overhearing a maternity nurse look at her newborn and say, "Gosh, I've never seen one like this before." The mom didn't know what the nurse meant, but it caused her great anxiety. For years, she continued wondering whether there was something wrong with her son. That one careless comment significantly hindered the mom's attachment.

## Parents' Attachments to Their Own Parents

Whether we like it or not, the way our own parents treated us usually affects how we parent our children. If a new mom had a traumatic birth when she was born or perhaps had an insecure attachment with her own mother, it could make her pregnancy, birth, and attachment to her own baby more difficult. The good news is that this past legacy can be dramatically changed when new parents remember how their own parents emotionally hurt them and consciously work to create relationships with their own infants that are more positive. "Research in the field of child development has demonstrated that a child's security of attachment to parents is strongly connected to the parents' understanding of their [own] early-life experiences."[67]

So, if you had a difficult childhood and try your best to remember how you were hurt, the chance of repeating this with your own youngsters becomes greatly reduced. Some therapists practice a new type of treatment with pregnant couples called "prenatal bonding" that can help heal parents' own attachment wounds in order to improve their attachments to their unborn babies.[68] The love hormones that are available in both the mother's and father's bodies and brains at the time of birth create a very favorable opportunity for beginning this parent-infant relationship in a new and loving way. While no one can ever be a perfect parent, each birth provides us with a fresh beginning and a chance to break the cycle of painful parent-child relationships from past generations. At the birth of your own baby, an opportunity to have the parent-child relationship you always wanted suddenly becomes available to you in a new form.

## Postpartum Mood Disorder

Most new mothers (fifty to eighty percent) experience a form of depression, called the "baby blues," within the first ten days after childbirth while their hormones are making dramatic shifts. Twenty percent of mothers have symptoms that continue past these first couple of weeks or that emerge at any time during the first year after the birth. The term postpartum mood disorder (PMD) is now often used, rather than that of postpartum depression, because the problematic symptoms are not always depression, but can be anxiety, insomnia, confusion, feelings of panic, obsessive-compulsive behavior, and disturbing intrusive thoughts or fears. If a woman was depressed or anxious during her pregnancy or had previous mood disorder episodes, she may be more prone to such problems during the postpartum months. Other risk factors include stress, isolation, a family history of depression, anxiety, bipolar illness, or a reaction to newly-taken birth control hormones.[69] It is important to point out that PMD is a very different disorder from postpartum psychosis, in which one's symptoms could include delusions, suspiciousness, auditory or visual hallucinations, incoherent speech, and grossly disorganized behavior, such as denial of the birth.

While PMD is most likely biochemically triggered, a lack of sleep and social support significantly contribute to its manifestation. In the peaceful cultures where a great deal of nurturing is given to women during their pregnancies and postpartum months, there is significantly less PMD. Along with emotional support, women recover more quickly when they get direct hands-on help with household chores and care of the baby. Feeling guilty, not asking for help, not taking breaks from the baby, and not taking care of her own needs can contribute to making the new mom's symptoms worse and more prolonged.

When a woman experiences a postpartum mood disorder, it does not mean that she will always feel this way, she is failing as a mom, or that she will never attach to her baby. While challenging, it is a temporary condition and all of the symptoms subside over time. Some treatments that have proven helpful are: exercise, diet, counseling, support groups, spiritual practice, natural remedies, and medication. Medication (some are even okay to use while breastfeeding) can be very helpful in alleviating the symptoms, as is having the support of other women, especially those who have experienced such a postpartum difficulty themselves. Trying to keep the communication open with her partner and seeking support from those who are sensitive, understanding, and not critical also contribute to helping a new mom's postpartum symptoms subside.[70]

A mood disorder after the birth of her baby can interfere with a new mother's ability to feel close to her baby, hindering early attachment, and also impacting the baby's ability to interact positively with his mom. If a mom's face is consistently sad or mad, an infant will begin looking away rather than into the mother's eyes. Nevertheless, with some help, moms who experience postpartum mood disorders can become wonderfully engaged mothers and develop strong loving attachments with their babies.

## Fear of Spoiling

One of the saddest factors that often inhibits attachment is the completely erroneous fear that if a parent gives the baby too much love and attention, the baby will become "spoiled." I have heard parents talk about how they fought their instincts and forced themselves not to offer comfort or respond to their baby's cries because they thought it would be better for their baby. One of the most fundamental aspects of parenting that must be understood is that *an infant cannot be spoiled by too much attention or affection.* If there can only be one "take home" message from this book, this one should be at the top of the list.

Lack of attention is what damages an infant and the parent's relationship with that infant. When babies cry, they are responding to internal discomforts that they need the help of a caregiver to meet because infants are completely incapable of meeting any of their own needs. For the first year to eighteen months of life, babies benefit greatly from having all their needs met as soon as possible. I believe that not responding to infants teaches them that they are not worthy of being cared for and not to be compassionate to others' cries for help. If a mother can "close her ears" to her infant's pain, she is teaching that "closing the door" to the pain of others is acceptable or even advisable. Feelings of abandonment, a lack of trust, and learning not to ask for help or respond compassionately to others are lessons that get recorded in the heart and preverbal subconscious mind. Infants cannot "learn to self-calm" by being left alone when crying. The opposite is true: babies who are held and comforted during their first year of life are much better at self-calming when older. Remember, independence comes from security, and security comes from having physical and psychological needs met when infants are completely dependent.

A baby's brain does not come equipped with the ability to learn how to behave appropriately. Babies do not have the ability to outsmart or manipulate, despite what some people mistakenly believe. It is not until fourteen and eighteen months of age that babies' brains become ready to understand such complex cause and effect interconnections. At that age, toddlers are becoming ready to learn socially acceptable behaviors, and at that point, parents should start setting limits and teaching socially appropriate behavior. Infancy, however, is solely a time of learning about love and trust, which, when given, creates a strong foundation from which an open-hearted, trusting, and lovable child can develop (see photo 14).

# CHAPTER 4

# Parenting Styles
# in the United States

*Education should be in harmony with the child's essentially kind nature.*
*The most important element is that children be raised in a climate*
*of love and tenderness.*

—The Dalai Lama

The way we parent our children is typically learned early in life from the way we are parented as children. Most of our early parenting is recorded in our subconscious minds since we go through three years of being parented before we can describe it in words and seven years before we can process this information logically. The old saying that "kids do as we do, not as we say" is very accurate. Modeling adult behavior is the most powerful way that children learn, and the majority of our lifetime behaviors are learned before we are six years old. Research has shown that the way a preschooler treats her dolls is highly predictive of how she will later mother her children. In one experimental study, preschool children were exposed to adults being aggressive toward certain dolls; the kids were later observed to be aggressive toward those very same dolls.[1] Unless we deliberately attempt to change negatively ingrained parenting practices, we will likely repeat those same behaviors with our own children, especially when angry or stressed, once our subconscious reactions take over. All parents can probably relate to those shocking inner-voice moments of "Whoa, I can't believe I just did that, I promised myself I would *never* do that to my kids!"

Sociology researcher Brené Brown PhD, after reviewing thousands of personal stories related to feelings of shame and inadequacy, discovered that a sense of "worthiness" is the variable that separates individuals who have feelings of being loveable and belonging from those who constantly struggle in relationships. Dr. Brown believes that the most essential ingre-

71

---

### Four Main Parenting Styles

- Authoritarian
- Inconsistent
- Permissive
- Relational

---

dient to leading a happy life is the feeling of being loveable. She found that what keeps people from connecting with others is usually fear that they are not worthy of those relationships. Put simply, those who believe they are worthy of love are those who end up in strong loving relationships.[2] It is my belief that self-worth develops very early in life and is related to the way babies are welcomed during their gestations, births, and first attempts at crying out for attention. Feelings of self-worth develop more positively if the cries of infants and young children are answered with care and concern rather than resentment or neglect. How children are parented from the beginning of life either promotes inner beliefs that they are worthy of attention, affection, belonging, and love or leaves them feeling unlovable with a foundation of self-doubt, fear, and shame.

As a psychologist, I have heard heartbreaking stories from clients with tears streaming down their faces as they recount childhood memories of being physically and/or emotionally wounded by their parents. I've even known clients who purposely chose not to have children because they were afraid of repeating the ways they had been hurt. I champion those who are willing to recall not only the helpful, but also the harmful parenting they received; remembering both these extremes is the only way healthier parenting styles can evolve. Our memories can help us replicate those parenting practices that helped us become confident, resilient, compassionate, and emotionally healthy, while consciously avoiding those that were damaging to our self-esteem, trust, and fear of being close to others.

So, what are the models for parenting in our culture that determine the ways we treat our children? The four main parenting styles currently used in the US are referred to as:

Authoritarian, Inconsistent, Permissive, and what I call Relational.

## Four Main Parenting Styles

### Authoritarian Parenting

Authoritarian Parenting has been historically promoted in the United States and other parts of the world for many generations. With Authoritarian Parenting, there is a strongly held conviction that parents should limit affection and strictly control their children's behavior. Dr. John B. Watson's 1928 book, *Psychological Care of Infant and Child,* told parents, "Never, never kiss your child . . . . Never hold it in your lap. Never rock its carriage."[3] Authoritarian parents are warned that being too affectionate or responding quickly to their baby's cries will result in whiny, demanding children. Reduced response to crying infants is advocated due to the false belief that it will help children become emotionally stronger and independent.

Such parenting has rigid rules as to what a parent should and should not do. It does not take into account individual differences between infants or encourage parents to listen to their own feelings concerning what their child may need at a particular moment in his ever-changing body and mind. Parents are convinced that they should adhere to a strict four-hour time-regulated feeding schedule. Some mothers relate stories of painfully pacing outside their screaming infant's closed doors, often for hours, wringing their hands and anxiously watching the clock until they are "allowed" to pick up and feed their traumatized babies.

Authoritarian Parenting demands unquestioning obedience of toddlers and older children. It is believed that children are naturally disobedient and manipulative, needing to be treated unsympathetically and harshly. Adherence to the old "spare the rod, spoil the child" belief promotes the use of severe physical and emotional punishments to insure strict compliance. Professor Emeritus of Biology, Mary Clark PhD, who taught in England beginning in the mid-1950s recounts a common saying that she found disturbing: "Speak sharply to your little boy and scold him when he sneezes. He only does it to annoy, and since he knows it teases."[4]

Authoritarian mothers are expected to react immediately to inappropriate behavior by hitting the child with their hands or the nearest available object. At the same time it is commonly expected that the fathers will administer the harshest premeditated corporal punishments with paddles, belts, razor strops, and other instruments specifically used to inflict intense pain. Thus the ominous warning to naughty children is: "Wait until your father gets home."

Common also to this parenting model are frequent threats of physical harm if children don't obey. Such warnings as "You better do it before I count to three" or "Stop crying or I'll give you something to cry about," tend to create children who behave out of fear rather than a desire to cooperate. Some children will continue to misbehave until just before the number "three" is reached; they only change their behavior to avoid being punished, not because they want to gain parental approval, act appropriately, or have a guilty conscience.

Also included in Authoritarian Parenting is emotional wounding done verbally by shaming, blaming, or name-calling. Most of us know that condemning words can leave lifelong wounds, which challenge our core feelings of self-worth and lovability.

This type of punitive parenting is usually passed down from generation to generation: a person who is bullied and hit as a child is likely to bully and hit others, including his own children. What people raised by Authoritarian Parenting seem to remember most is that their parents were frightening, unpredictable, and would hurt them. The greatest lessons usually learned were: lying is often safer than telling the truth, become sneaky to avoid getting caught, and don't trust adults when they are angry. Fear, rather than sought after respect, is what the majority of folks raised with Authoritarian Parenting remember feeling in relation to their parents.

There are currently some popular Authoritarian Parenting programs in which parents are encouraged to use hands, belts, and other instruments for striking their children in attempts to control their behavior. One such Christian-based program is promoted in Michael and Debi Pearl's book *To Train Up A Child*. The Pearls' "No Greater Joy" ministry dictates that it is the parents' responsibility to control their children's will and demand total obedience. They support punishment by "thumping" a child and "switching" him with an instrument that will inflict pain without leaving bruises. The Pearls believe that a parent should train a child early, "before the need for discipline arises."[5] Some cases of severe child abuse and even death have resulted from parents following these practices.[6]

Another popular Authoritarian Parenting program that has gained considerable momentum is advocated in *On Becoming Babywise* by Gary Ezzo, first published in 1994.[7] Ezzo fosters the belief that parents should not be burdened by their children and need to use physical punishments to make them obey. Ezzo claims that by using the Babywise "Infant Management Plan," parents can "successfully and naturally help infants synchronize their feeding, wake-time, and nighttime sleep cycles." It promises "nighttime sleep, healthy babies, and rested mothers."[8] Ezzo's current popularity is associated with trying to teach infants by two months of age to sleep through the night. While toddlers do well when having some regularity in their daily lives, babies should never be expected to adhere to a rigidly enforced schedule. Infants do not have control of when they are hungry, wet, or able to fall asleep. Pediatrician Matthew Aney has discredited Ezzo's "parent directed feeding" strategy as causing breast milk failure, dehydration, poor weight gain, early weaning, and failure to thrive. Dr. Aney states that Ezzo's advice is in direct opposition to the American Academy of Pediatrics' recommendations on newborn feeding.[9] Ezzo, previously a Christian pastor, has tempered some of his early rigidity in parenting practices and now co-publishes with a pediatrician. He continues, however, to caution against the over-nurturing of newborns and advocates that babies be required to fit into their parents' lives, rather than parents adapting to their babies' needs. Healthcare professionals and prominent Christian leaders alike have been alarmed and have voiced concerns about Ezzo's parenting program.[10]

There are some infants who naturally "fit" more easily into a parent's desired feeding and sleeping schedule, while others require much more flexibility and take longer to settle into a family's routine. It is important to remember that one timetable does not work for all babies. While my son took long naps and slept through the night within a few months, my daughter's longest nap was about twenty minutes and she continued to wake up at least three times a night until she was three years old. It is critical during those early years for parents to be sensitive to their baby's individual needs; it pays off in the long run, as it helps youngsters develop trust in relationships. It is now known that lack of nurturing of a newborn is emotional starvation that can critically alter early brain development.[11] Research has demonstrated that children raised with Authoritarian Parenting are less motivated to please their parents and tend to be more withdrawn, angry, defiant, and lack self-control.[12]

## Inconsistent Parenting

Strict Authoritarian Parenting of past generations began to change with the baby boomers in 1946 due to the revolutionary parenting guide by Dr. Benjamin Spock, *The Common Sense Book of Baby and Child Care.* Instead of adhering to the inflexible authoritarian model of rigid rules that should be applied to all children, Spock urged parents to view their children as individuals and be more adaptable in meeting their needs. Dr. Spock coached parents to trust their "own common sense" as to what their babies needed, adding that "cuddling babies and bestowing affection on children would only make them happier and more secure."[13] Mothers were still encouraged, however, to consider their own convenience in creating an approximate four-hour feeding and sleeping schedule for their babies. While Dr. Spock's advice marked a turning point in the field of children's emotional health, parents, who themselves had been raised with an authoritarian approach, were often inconsistent in how they parented.

Inconsistent Parenting resulted from parents becoming confused as to what was best. They would sometimes respond to their crying baby, while at other times watched the clock until an appropriate number of hours had passed before answering their baby's cries. Parents often just reverted to the way they had been parented because they worried about "spoiling" their children.

This post-war era was also a time of increased medical intervention during hospitalized childbirths: laboring mothers were given heavy sedation, fathers were banned from labor and delivery, newborns were instantly removed and taken to a nursery, and formula rather than breastfeeding was strongly encouraged. All of these factors contributed to insecure parent-infant attachments and inconsistent parenting practices.

Parenting becomes inconsistent when a baby is held, fed, comforted, and cared for at certain times, but not at others. Lack of dependability on mom or dad in trying to meet their baby's needs interferes with the baby being able to relax and trust in these first most important relationships. Inability to trust leads to an insecure attachment that may be observed as either "ambivalent" (babies who cry a lot and are anxious about whether their needs will be met) or "avoidant" (babies who ignore, turn away, shut down). Insecure attachments can lead to later difficulties in problem solving, trusting oneself and others, empathy, worthiness, having healthy relationships, and regulating one's emotions (i.e. being able to control outbursts of anger).

The difference in how less closely connected American parents are with their infants compared to others in the world is shocking.

- A study done in 1972 reported that mothers in the US deliberately ignored forty-six percent of their babies' crying episodes during the first three months of life.[14]
- In my 1989 observations of parenting in Bali and a 1994 Korean study done by K. Lee,[15] the amount of time a baby spends alone at one month of age in Bali was zero percent, in Korea was 8.3 percent, and in the US was 67.5 percent.
- A 1992 study found that the US consistently stood out as *the only society* in which babies were routinely placed in their own beds and own rooms.[16]

The aversion to keeping a sleeping baby close to his parents continues currently in the US (See discussion on Co-Sleeping in Chapter 3). While tired mothers, especially those who are breastfeeding, find it much easier to sleep with their infants in the same bed or at least the same room, many feel guilty and often hide this natural maternal behavior. Inconsistency can arise when a mom feels anxiety, confusion, or guilt about her parenting; this can interfere with her ability to listen to her baby and trust herself in meeting his needs. Conflict and inconsistency can also arise between the two parents when they have differing beliefs as to what is best for their baby.

## What Ferberizing may be like for a baby . . .

Little four-month-old Logan is just blossoming into a content, trusting, and joyful baby. He has felt very comfortable at night sleeping in a crib in his parents' room and listening to their breathing when he arouses from sleep. His mommy and daddy always listen to his cries, are responsive to his physical needs, and give him lots of attention and affection. Suddenly one night, his crib is moved into another room, and when Logan wakes up, startled at being alone, he cries out. He feels great relief when his mommy comes into the room and speaks to him, but unexpectedly, she doesn't pick him up or even touch him. Logan is confused and cries louder, but his mommy just turns her back and walks out of the room. Shocked by this, he cries even louder, but no one comes to help him for a long time. At last, his daddy enters the room and offers some soothing words, but dad doesn't touch or pick up Logan either. As Logan begins to scream, very frightened by his parents' sudden change in behavior, he watches his daddy also turn and walk away from him. Now he is terrified, but it seems that the louder Logan cries, the longer it takes for one of his parents to come back into the room. Logan screams for what seems like forever, but still his parents refuse to pick him up and comfort him. Logan finally passes out from exhaustion, but that night his sense of safety and complete trust in his parents has been lost forever.

The concept of Ferberization, developed by Dr. Richard Ferber, is a currently popular Inconsistent Parenting practice that attempts to get babies to sleep for longer intervals at night. Parents who previously responded to their infant's cries are coached, when their baby is about four months of age, to suddenly stop providing physical comfort at night. Parents are told they can respond verbally to the baby, but not pick him up or give him any physical comfort.

This process is continued at progressively increasing intervals, with parents being told to wait five more minutes each time before returning to the crying baby's room.[17] While some babies may be ready to sleep for longer periods and will respond to such an approach by fussing for a few minutes and then quieting, most four-month-old babies will become extremely frightened by this sudden change in their parents' behavior and will scream loudly for help. An unanswered baby will eventually collapse into sleep, but at what price? At four months, a baby cannot understand that he is suddenly expected not to ask for help during the night or to know why he is comforted during the daytime, but not when it is dark. For some babies this type of cry-it-out approach can even be traumatic, leading to feelings of vulnerability, abandonment, numbing of emotional response (crying stops due to detachment and/or withdrawal), and insecurity in the relationship.[18] I have known babies who began anxiously clinging to their parents, crying more during the daytime, and becoming unable to relax into sleep even when suckling after their parents attempted to Ferberize them. Parents who are empathic to their baby's feelings will know if Feberizing is harmful their baby and should listen to their own feelings about it. Even Dr. Ferber is now clarifying that he never intended for parents to completely ignore their baby's nighttime cries.[19]

Researchers at Yale University and Harvard Medical School have discovered that the hormone cortisol, which is released in humans when they are overly stressed, can damage or even destroy neurons in babies' still developing brains. This neural toxin increases the potential for a lifetime of anxiety, learning difficulties, and problems with interpersonal relationships.[20] Is it worth risking all of this just to have a baby sleep longer during the night a few months earlier than he naturally would anyway? It's sort of like trying to get a nine-month-old to walk instead of waiting until he does it on his own at twelve months.

Dr. Spock revolutionized parenting by beginning to enlighten parents to the dangers of being authoritarian, and he attempted to move them toward more compassionate care of their children. Clearly, further change in the direction of more consistent responsive parenting is needed. Being able to love and to feel loved is a primal human need. So many people, however, are fearful of love because they were not able to trust in a dependable, loving relationship from the very beginning of life.

To avoid this disconnect, I believe in fostering an approach that I call the "love triangle": when one feels loved, then one can trust, and when one can trust, then one can be loving.

## Permissive Parenting

Permissive or overindulgent parents are at the opposite end of the continuum from authoritarian parents. Permissive parents are nondirective, very lenient, and exceedingly responsive to their children's needs and desires. When babies receive this kind of consistent loving care, they grow feelings of self-worth and lovability. At about eighteen months of age, however, toddlers begin to need clear direction, limit setting, and help with learning self-control. Some well-meaning, nurturing parents don't understand that infants' developmental needs are very different from those of toddlers.

When parents continue being excessively indulgent with toddlers and older children, this is where the "spoiled child" syndrome can begin to emerge. Toddlers raised without clear expectations as to how they should behave can end up controlling the entire family. Permissive parents often ignore demanding and inconsiderate behavior, tending to give in to their child's increasingly persistent demands. These parents are inclined to plead, bribe, and make requests into questions often ending with an "OK?" Such as, "Your toys need to be picked up, OK?" Children raised this way don't learn to listen and respect the requests of adults. They can become extremely self-centered, lack respect for others' needs, expect to always get their own way, and blame others for their mistakes. This self-absorbed behavior can cause kids considerable difficulty with peers and in later social relationships.[21]

In the extreme, when parents don't set age-appropriate limits to keep their children physically and emotionally safe, Permissive Parenting can even become neglectful parenting. Parents become neglectful when they believe their child is more able to make knowledgeable decisions and use mature judgment than she is capable of doing. When children are mentally advanced and "talk smart," adults often believe they are therefore more emotionally mature, but a child's emotional age is actually the same as her age in years, not her mental age. This also can cause kids a great deal of anxiety because they are really too young to handle their parents' expectations. When parenting is too permissive, children often begin challenging authority figures at school and in other life situations, believing they are always right. Without respect for adult mentors, these kids can later lack self-control, be unable to learn from negative experiences, become aimless, and be more prone to alienation and drug use.[22]

## Relational Parenting

*Relational* is my term for the type of parenting that is most similar to that used in the peaceful cultures. Relational parents respond to children's feelings, offer children reasonable choices, and exercise parental control without being overbearing. The term Autho*ritative* Parenting, not to be confused with Autho*ritarian* Parenting, has also been used to describe this type of parenting. The primary goal of Relational Parenting is to foster a close parent-child relationship while helping children become confident, self-monitoring, and socially well-adjusted. Children are treated with a great deal of affection and compassion, but also with clear limits and expectations of self-control and compliance. Relational parents tend to promote empathy and altruism by helping their children become aware of other people's feelings and how their behavior affects others.[23] Not wanting their children to just become "pleasers," always accommodating, they teach their children to create a healthy balance between their own and others' needs.

Compassion in our children develops from being treated with kindness when they are young. Your baby will be trying to form a relationship with you from the minute she is born. Because babies are completely helpless, they are very desperate to communicate. If you watch your baby's body language, the cues as to what she needs get clearer and clearer. When you respond to a baby's subtle communications, a trusting relationship begins to develop: the baby can relax, knowing she is safe, listened to, and cared for. A content baby is able to spend her time learning new things, while a baby who is fearful for her basic survival is focused solely on that. If a baby doesn't feel safe, she will cry louder and longer trying to get someone

---

### Compassion for Others

Emily, at age ten, responded to an unsettling event in Nepal very differently than we, her parents, did. While walking down a city street filled with people, cars, and roaming animals, we tried to scoot past a huge pig just as he began to pee. All the adults on the street began to squeal and curse at the pig as urine splashed over our shoes and pant legs. Emily merely stepped out of the spray and kindly proclaimed, "Wow, I bet he feels lots better; he really had to go."

---

to listen, even though this may further distance her parents. Psychologist Mary Ainsworth found that American mothers who were sensitive to their infants' needs and responded promptly tended to have infants who were the most securely attached. These babies cried less and were more easily quieted when they did cry.[24] Gabor Maté, MD, an internationally-known supporter of close parent-child relationships, states that, "It is in their relationship, with us that our children will reach their developmental destiny of becoming independent, self-motivated, and mature beings valuing their own self-worth and mindful of the feelings, rights, and human dignity of others."[25]

Three types of Relational Parenting, which will be described in more detail, are Attachment Parenting, Connection Parenting, and Mindful Parenting.

The best-known Relational Parenting program is the American-based *Attachment Parenting* movement by William and Martha Sears. The international mission of the Sears is "to educate and support all parents in raising secure, joyful, and empathic children in order to strengthen families and create a more compassionate world."[26] Attachment Parenting has seven main principles, "The 7 Baby B's," that stress the importance of the following parenting practices: Birth and Bonding experiences, responsive Breastfeeding, Baby Wearing as much as possible, Bedding Close to the Baby to minimize nighttime separation anxiety, Belief in the Language of Baby's Cries as communications of need, Beware of Baby Trainers that promote detachment, and Balance of parents' needs with babies' needs.[27]

---

### Attachment Parenting's 7 Baby B's

- Birth and Bonding
- Breastfeeding
- Baby Wearing
- Bedding Close to the Baby
- Belief in the Language of Baby Cries
- Beware of Baby Trainers
- Balance

---

It is striking to notice how similar the first five Baby Bs are to the Global Practices that Increase Attachment that I have observed throughout the world (Chapter 3). The Sears' addition of the sixth principle, "Beware of Baby Trainers," refers to the current Authoritarian Parenting programs mentioned earlier in this chapter. The seventh principle, "Balance," is vitally important because it helps parents remember to balance the baby's needs with those of other children in the family and also the parents' own needs. In attempts to meet a baby's needs, along with those of their other children, jobs, and home, some dedicated parents forget to care for themselves and their own relationships. This lack of self-care can quickly lead to exhausted, depressed parents, and stressed marriages. It is essential to balance the baby's needs with those of others in the family.

Parenting is one of the very few 24/7 jobs in the world, and it is virtually impossible to instantly meet every need that your baby will have. Keep in mind that most important is a parent's overall attitude. Letting your baby or older child know you hear him crying out for help by answering with, "Sorry, I can't come right now, but will be there as soon as I can," conveys that you care, while helping you also take care of other needs, including your own.

The Sears' *Attachment Parenting* has specific suggestions for helping babies sleep longer during the night. Their book *The No-Cry Sleep Solution: Gentle Ways to Help Your Baby Sleep Through the Night* offers baby-friendly advice and is a welcome alternative to Ferberizing. The Sears have also written books that use their attachment principles to help with such issues as birth, breastfeeding, fussy babies, nighttime parenting, family nutrition, medical information, and becoming a new father.

Another excellent Relational Parenting program is *Connection Parenting: Parenting Through Connection Instead of Coercion, Through Love Instead of Fear* by Pam Leo. Leo has spent many decades as a childcare provider and gives workshops to parents and professionals concerning children's needs. Her basic belief is that youngsters require a consistent, loving connection with at least one adult in order to thrive physically, psychologically, emotionally, and spiritually.[28] Leo notes that because of our busy modern lives, babies beginning at twelve weeks of age often spend the majority of their waking hours away from parents. She suggests that these babies have unmet early needs that result in countless behavioral and emotional problems later in childhood. Leo adds, "The level of cooperation parents get from their children is usually equal to the level of connection children feel with their parents."[29] Because behavior is the way children communicate their needs, parents are cautioned not to control or change children's misbehavior until the cause for it is clearly understood. Leo believes, and I agree, that if a child is feeling a strong connection with his caregiver, he will want to please that adult and behave cooperatively. Dr. Maté offers the same opinion: "A child must be receptive if we are to succeed in nurturing, comforting, guiding, and directing her . . . . For a child to be open to being parented by an adult, he must be actively attaching to that adult, be wanting contact and closeness with him."[30]

So, if the relationship with your child is stressed, it is important to work on repairing the relationship first, and your child will most likely become more compliant as a result. Isn't that true in all our relationships? When we feel close to someone, aren't we much more positive and cooperative with him? Children are no different.

Leo describes connection as a feeling of being loved and listened to, while disconnection results in feelings of hurt and anger from being misunderstood or disregarded. Since babies and young children are not able to communicate verbally, they communicate by acting out their needs: this is aptly termed "acting-out behavior." A strongly held belief of my child-psychologist mentor, Dr. Vivian Olum, which has served me well over the years, is that *the person in the family acting least loveable at any given moment is usually the one needing the most!* Leo hopes parents can realize that when children's needs are met, they usually become delightful little kids. People who were not parented this way may question these tactics. But as Oprah Winfrey, quoted by Leo, says, "We did the best with what we knew; now we know more, so we can do better."[31]

Mindful Parenting is my own blend of relational parenting practices fine-tuned from decades of observing parents around the world, developing techniques that have worked well for clients, and those that have been successful with my own kids. Mindful Parenting For Toddlers and Young Children, which includes validating children's feelings and using a unique method of discipline called Time-In that teaches self-control, will be described in Chapter 5.

Those who use parenting methods at either end of the continuum, by being overly controlling or overly permissive, tend to have children with difficulties in self-regulation, interpersonal relationships, and overall contentment in life. A recent study of the long-term impact on teenagers resulting from differing parenting styles found that Authoritarian parents who were low on warmth but high on accountability had teens whose risk of participating in heavy alcohol drinking was *more than double* that of the Relational parenting group. Permissive parents who were high in warmth but low in accountability had teens who were *three times more likely* to participate in heavy drinking. Relational parents who were high in both warmth and expectations of accountability raised teens who were *the least* prone to heavy drinking.[32]

Relational Parenting promotes the formation of secure attachments between parents and children. The incredible lifelong benefits for children who have a securely-attached relationship during the first two years of life are independence, self-reliance, social responsibility, resilience in times of stress, the ability to self-calm, increased self-esteem, greater compassion toward others, and being comfortable with intimacy.[33] Research studies continually reveal that closely connected relationships based on mutual respect from very early in life are essential to the well-being of humans.

Simply said, it is much more important what you do *with* your children than what you do *to* your children.

## Punishment vs. Discipline

Authoritarian Parenting has left many generations of people feeling emotionally wounded and disconnected from their parents. It was common for children in the past not to have their feelings understood or respected. They were punished by being slapped, spanked, hit with objects, put in rooms alone while crying, shamed, blamed, disregarded, belittled, and often given consequences totally unrelated to their behavior. When remembering punishments that hurt them physically and emotionally, most people recall that it resulted in them becoming sneaky, angry, dishonest, disconnected, distrustful, depressed, and ultimately fearful of their parents. It is just not in our nature to feel trust and love toward someone who hurts us. While most people know that their parents did the best job they could with the knowledge and resources they had, now that we know what kids truly need, we have an opportunity to do it very differently.

When parents use painful punishments, they can stop the undesirable behavior in the moment, but the child, likely, will become more resentful and reluctant to please, developing instead more devious ways to avoid being caught. At the same time, modern parents who have strong connections with their children worry about how they can set limits on inappropriate behavior without wounding those relationships or dampening their children's spirits. This is where discipline, rather than punishment, is the answer. It is critical to understand the difference between punishment and discipline!

The definition of *punishment* is "to cause pain, loss, or suffering,"[34] while *discipline* (which comes from the word disciple) means "to instruct or educate; training that develops self-control, character, and orderly conduct."[35] The latter is surely the goal of most parents.

Our tragic history of child maltreatment, which followed the historical belief that children are born immoral and will be further "spoiled" if not subjected to painful punishments, has clearly been proven wrong.

Research findings from neuroscience, developmental psychology, biology, and anthropology are all converging with clear evidence that abuse, neglect, and lack of nurturing are what damage a child. Extensive research has shown that there is a direct connection between corporal punishment of children and their later aggressive or violent behavior as teenagers and adults.[36] Australian psychologist Robin Grille also does research on parenting practices that can help create a more peaceful world. According to his findings, "The human brain and heart that are met primarily with empathy in the critical early years cannot and will not grow to choose a violent or selfish life."[37]

As in the peaceful cultures, many other countries have for decades outlawed all forms of violence against children, including that which is used to force obedience. In 1958, Sweden was the first to ban corporal punishment in schools, followed in 1979 with a law that prohibited parental use of physical punishments or other humiliating treatments with children.[38] The United Nations Committee on the Rights of the Child has since 1996 encouraged all countries to outlaw the corporal punishment of children. Outright bans against physical punishment of children in all settings (home, school, day care, etc.) currently exist in thirty-three countries: Albania, Austria, Bulgaria, Congo, Costa Rica, Croatia, Cyprus, Denmark, Finland, Germany, Greece, Honduras, Hungary, Iceland, Israel, Kenya, Latvia, Liechtenstein, Luxembourg, Netherlands, New Zealand, Norway, Poland, Portugal, Republic of Moldova, Romania, South Sudan, Spain, Togo, Tunisia, Ukraine, Uruguay, and Venezuela. Governments in the following forty-nine countries have made commitments to develop laws that would end all legalized aggressive treatment of children: Afghanistan, Algeria, Armenia, Azerbaijan, Bangladesh, Belize, Bhutan, Bolivia, Brazil, Burkina Faso, Cape Verde, Chad, Ecuador, El Salvador, Estonia, India, Lithuania, Maldives, Mauritius, Mongolia, Montenegro, Morocco, Nepal, Nicaragua, Niger, Pakistan, Palau, Panama, Papua New Guinea, Peru, Philippines, Samoa, San Marino, São Tomé and Principe, Serbia, Slovakia, Slovenia, South Africa, Sri Lanka, Tajikistan, Macedonia, Thailand, Timor-Leste, Turkey, Turkmenistan, Uganda, Zambia, and Zimbabwe.[39] It is commendable that so many countries have outlawed the infliction of pain on children as a basic human rights issue. In 2013,

5.4 percent of all children on the earth were lawfully protected from any form of corporal punishment and when all those countries committed to making such laws are able to achieve full prohibition, 45.9 percent of the global child population will be safe from painfully cruel treatment.[40] In order to avoid having societies swing from Authoritarian to overly Permissive Parenting, it is important that parents be educated in clear limit setting with expectations of compliance beginning in toddlerhood using a method such as Time-In, which is discussed in the following chapter.

While corporal punishment in US schools has been banned in thirty-one states and Washington, DC, we have not yet had one state able to successfully ban the striking of children by their parents as long as it doesn't leave a bruise or cause a fracture.[41] How has the US lagged so far behind numerous other countries in realizing that hitting a child is just as wrong as hitting an adult? If someone strikes an adult, it is considered an illegal assault; but somehow, hitting a defenseless child is still considered acceptable by some people. Hopefully, the spanking of children will one day be recognized throughout the world as unnecessary and harmful in the same way as beating women is now outlawed in most cultures.

Decades ago I decided that if I saw a child was being hurt, it would be my duty to intervene. Since then, I have approached many angry, overwhelmed parents with kind words such as, "I know how hard parenting can be. It looks like you could use some support." I am usually met with the angry reply, "This is none of your business!" To which I have found the best response to be, "Well, actually, since you are doing this in front of me, it is my business, and if anyone was hitting you in front of me, I would also try to stop them." A look of surprise usually crosses the distressed parents' faces, and the hitting almost always stops. I believe that this intervention often triggers memories of how it felt to be slapped as children and maybe even wishes that someone would have intervened when adults were hurting them. Hopefully, it plants a seed of awareness in parents' minds that hitting their children is no more okay than it was for someone to hit them.

Every parent loses her temper when pushed beyond the limits of her patience. At these times, the parent (whose heart is racing and blood pressure peaking) will usually lash out verbally at first; but if the child's misbehavior continues, she will react most likely in the same way she was treated by her parents. With a previous commitment not to inflict harm on her child, however, she could try a different tactic. If such an incident occurs at home or in a place where it is safe to leave the child alone, this would be an excellent time for the mom to take a "time-out" of her own. She could say something like, "Mommy really needs a break right now." Going outside for a breather (counting to ten and/or taking some deep breaths really does help) or going into the bathroom and locking the door could give her the brief respite she needs to consider some options. I certainly resorted to such self-imposed "time-outs" when my children were youngsters and teens. I've been told that Balinese parents even sometimes resort to controlling toddlers by telling them that ghosts or evil spirits will get them if they don't behave. Think how much better it would be if parents could just take "time-outs" rather than saying or doing something that inflicted physical or emotional injury on their children. Using this type of self-control also serves as an excellent model of anger management for children to observe.

## Push the Refresh Button

Parenting is by far the most complex, confusing, challenging, and ever-changing job anyone will ever encounter. While most parents want to do the best job they can to help their children grow up happily well adjusted, they are frequently bewildered when their children misbehave, and can often resort to actions they later regret. It is never possible to parent without making mistakes. When you've done something that creates hurt and distance between you and your child, the most important parenting tip to remember is *always reconnect with your child as soon as possible.*

Rather than just feeling guilty when you regrettably lash out at your children, a simple apology can not only repair the relationship (and trust me, it is never too late), but helps kids know that all people, even their parents, make mistakes. Reconnecting also helps teach children how to "push the refresh button" in their own relationships when a disconnect occurs.

Although at times your parents may have treated you in ways that left some emotional scars, they most likely did what they thought best or parented you in the way they, themselves, had been parented. Remembering your pain, resentment, and feelings of disconnection from your own parents and desiring to parent differently is admirable. However, along with not blaming yourself too harshly for making parenting mistakes, you may also find it valuable at some point to stop blaming your own parents. After becoming a parent, a much better understanding develops as to just how overwhelmingly complex this job really is. Such new awareness can give you greater sympathy and acceptance for your own parents. It offers a fresh opportunity to heal old wounds and help you reconnect with them in new ways. This act of forgiveness will also allow your children to have much closer relationships with their grandparents.

In most of the world, parenting is done with a great deal of extended family support. While Hilary Clinton was definitely right that it indeed "takes a village" to raise a child, [42] first and foremost, it takes a family. This doesn't need to look like the traditional dad, mom, and two kids, but it does need to be a close loving group of people who spend time with and watch out for each child's well-being. This "family" needs to be individuals who are committed to love and care for the children throughout their child and teen years. Building this kind of support is one of the greatest gifts you can give your children; nothing can be more welcome than having loving grandparents and extended family members in your children's lives to help carry the load and share the joys.

# CHAPTER 5

# Mindful Parenting for Toddlers and Young Children

*The things that matter most in our lives are not fantastic or grand.*
*They are the moments when we touch one another.*
—Jack Kornfield

The peaceful cultures believe that all babies are born with a golden core of pure goodness. Balinese parenting best illustrates my own unique blend of Mindful Parenting practices with its acceptance that all children have a desire to be cooperative and can be encouraged to make good choices when parents help them "listen-inside" to their essentially agreeable nature and help them become the people they are meant to be. Mindful Parenting incorporates lessons I've learned from peaceful cultures along with being a mother and psychologist helping grow delightfully kind-hearted children with a high degree of self-control.

Mindful Parenting requires parents to be attentive and responsive to their children's needs, with the fundamental goal of maintaining close, mutually-compassionate relationships. Nurturing newborns using the Mindful Parenting of Infants techniques described in Chapter 3 creates a foundation that helps babies blossom into trusting, content, and loving toddlers. *I have consistently observed that the parental love-bond, which develops in the first eighteen months of a baby's life, is what later helps a toddler and older child be willing to cooperate with parents' requests and limits on inappropriate behavior.* Self-control and the development of a conscience begin with the toddler not wanting the beloved parent to be angry with him. If your child lacks the desire to please you (or another attached caregiver), he will have no reason to deny his own wishes, becoming a child who requires someone else to intervene repeatedly to control his misbehavior. While an intimate relationship between you and your child can be strongly shaped in the first eighteen months, navigating the next few years in a positive way will help you maintain a close connection as your child gets older.

Mindful Parenting as seen with Balinese parents involves helping toddlers become *mindful* of their own behavior. The time between one-and-a-half and three-and-a-half years of age is the stage in which toddlers:

- Acquire a conscience
- Develop self-control
- Learn to regulate their emotions
- Build socially appropriate behaviors

Many Americans refer to these years as the "terrible twos" and "trying threes," because this stage of development definitely requires new parenting skills. Parents often worry about how to set limits and teach their child to behave appropriately without squashing their child's will or damaging their relationships. Some parents, who have been very nurturing with their infants, suddenly switch to Authoritarian Parenting with their toddlers. Other parents remember how they were physically hurt by harsh punishments and felt frightened by their parents' anger, so they resort to overly Permissive Parenting. Either extreme leads to a less than optimal outcome.

I guarantee that toddlers can become well-socialized without any damage to their bodies, psyches, or your relationships with them when you follow these three principles of Mindful Parenting:

- Validate your toddler's feelings
- Communicate clearly what behavior you expect
- Use firm but fair discipline (not punishment) for uncooperative behavior

These three parenting practices can make the toddler years an enjoyable time for everyone in the family. For over thirty-five years, I have taught hundreds of parents these Mindful Parenting practices for toddlers. Feedback from parents has convinced me that these methods truly support parents in maintaining close loving relationships with their youngsters while helping them develop into well-behaved enjoyable children.

## Validating Feelings

At about eighteen months of age, it is important to assist toddlers in understanding their feelings and learning to express them in socially appropriate ways. Parents who explain what feelings are and good ways to express them help kids develop a type of emotional intelligence, which makes them more self-aware and empathetic toward others. Just as we offer names for objects when toddlers begin to speak, it is also important to help them identify their four basic feelings: *glad, sad, mad, and scared.*[1]

Please don't try to stop children from expressing their feelings or communicate to them that certain feelings are bad. Instead, teach children to listen to what their feelings are telling them. All of your children's feelings give them information that is important in helping them understand themselves. Feelings are their emotional GPS, directing them toward life experiences that are right for them and away from those they should avoid. Feelings tell them what brings them pleasure and pain, whom they can trust, what feels safe, and what should be avoided because it feels dangerous. Parents in peaceful cultures always respond to crying children with attempts to understand and offer comfort. I was disappointed, however, to discover that in Bali, children are often distracted from their sad feelings by being given sweets, and laughter is used to "cheer them up." The Balinese rightfully believe that when people get "stuck" in depression it reduces their ability to see available options that can help them move out of their sadness. While this is true for adults, toddlers rarely get stuck in a feeling since they instinctively know how to express them. When toddlers are glad, they smile, giggle, and laugh; when sad, they cry; if mad, they have what most call a "meltdown" or "tantrum," hitting, kicking, and screaming until they completely de-stress; and when scared, they run to someone they trust for safety and comfort. Toddlers who are encouraged to understand and express their feelings have a valuable resource that helps guide them through life.

In families where toddlers are shamed or punished for certain feelings, they will either start acting out or hiding those feelings, somewhere between the ages of three and five. Aptly referred to as "acting-out behavior," this is a toddler's attempt to show how and why he is upset. When children try to hide feelings it's harder to know what's bothering them. The feelings don't just go away, but usually get expressed indirectly, in ways that are irritating or confusing. For example:

- An angry child who is punished for feeling mad may start being mean to the family dog or become aggressive, bullying the kids at school.
- A sad child shamed for crying may become a constant whiner or withdraw into thumb sucking and TV watching.
- A scared toddler may have a hard time going to bed at night or begin waking up with nightmares. If not comforted and reassured, this child could develop separation anxiety, suddenly becoming terrified to be left at the preschool that he previously loved attending.

A child who tries to be very accommodating may get so adept at hiding feelings her parents don't like to witness that she may even learn to hide them from herself, causing lots of personal distress later in life. Examples of this that I have observed as a psychologist are:

- A young woman who lost her internal GPS as a very compliant little girl always deferred to others for direction. When asked how she felt about certain life experiences, she would look confused and respond with, "I don't know, how should I feel about that?"
- A preteen was once brought to see me because he repeatedly put himself in extremely dangerous situations. Upon questioning this behavior, he proudly proclaimed, "I've learned how never to feel afraid of anything!"

Parents who were taught as children not to express certain feelings may have difficulty supporting those emotions in their toddlers. It is common for parents to tell their children they are being "good" when they are happy and "bad" when they are mad, sad, or even scared. Although some feelings are more pleasant to witness than others, all feelings are important and none of them are "bad." Behavior can be unacceptable, but feelings are merely internal indicators as to how each of us as unique individuals experience the world. Just as paying attention to your own feelings helps you understand yourself, listening to your child's emotions can help you understand your child. Once you understand your child's feelings, you can help your child "listen inside" to identify those feelings, help her learn to express them in acceptable ways, and teach her how to use feelings as a guide to make choices that are right for her. Our feelings are our direct pathways to living a safe, happy, self-directed life.

In peaceful cultures it is believed that parents modeling and explaining how to express feelings is the best way for toddlers to learn culturally acceptable ways to deal with them. While American parents sometimes punish overwhelmed toddlers for having a "temper tantrum," parents in the peaceful cultures would be more likely to try to offer support and comfort. It helps to understand that these "meltdowns" are the way that toddlers "unstress" when they feel overwhelmed, and unstressing is an extremely healthy way of releasing tension! Toddlers *are not doing this to manipulate* or cause suffering for their parents; they have simply been overcome with frustration or anger. (I often wish that teens and adults had harmless ways of unstressing like toddlers do, rather than some of their commonly used damaging and addictive choices.) It is important for parents to teach their children not to hurt themselves or anyone else when they are unstressing, without causing their kids to feel badly for having such intense feelings.

In our culture, some feelings seem to be gender specific. Boys are frequently shamed for expressing sad or scared feelings, being called crybabies or sissies, while girls are often taught that nice little girls shouldn't yell or express anger. Blocking any of the four basic feelings, glad, sad, mad or scared, can lead to later emotional distress such as withdrawal, depression, anxiety, aggression, risk taking, substance abuse, and stress-related illnesses. Invalidating our children's feelings leads to confusion, self-doubt, and an erosion of self-esteem. On the other hand, when we validate their feelings, we help them trust their own inner voices and believe

## How parents can offer support and comfort to a toddler with intensely angry feelings

Maya is having a hard day. She has just learned to walk and is finally able to get to all those interesting things she has been looking at for the past year. As soon as she attempts to explore these treasures, however, each one is either suddenly removed from her reach or she is told sternly not to touch it. Maya, unable to cope with one more disappointment, falls to the floor screaming loudly and kicking the carpet. Maya's mom calmly sits near her toddler and reassures her that Mommy knows how frustrating it must be not to touch all those things, and that it is good that she is getting her mad out without hurting anyone or anything. Although Maya's mom still won't let Maya play with the untouchables, just having her feelings validated in this way helps Maya unstress, recover more quickly, and retreat to her mom's lap for some comfort and reassurance. Rather than being punished for becoming angry, Maya's mom helped Maya express her anger safely all the way through to recovery. The relationship between Maya and her mom even feels closer because Maya feels understood.

in themselves. In order to help your children respect and express their feelings it is usually important for parents to review their own emotional upbringing.

How did your parents react when you were glad, sad, mad, or scared? Were there particular feelings that you were shamed or punished for expressing? How did your parents' responses cause you feel? How do you wish they had responded? The answers to these questions may make it easier to understand how you want to react to your own children's feelings. Helping them understand their glad, sad, mad, and scared feelings and express them in healthy ways will serve them well throughout their lives along with deepening their trust in you as someone with whom they can share their emotions.

## Glad, Sad, Mad, and Scared

- *Glad* or happy is a feeling that most parents enjoy and welcome unless a child gets overly noisy or rambunctious. Champion your children's joy and direct them outside or into another room if it is disturbing, but let them have fun. Laughing and playing are fantastic ways to unstress.
- When *sad,* humans have a wonderfully adapted internal mechanism that automatically helps to remove sadness from our bodies; it's called crying. We are one of only a few mammals that cry tears. In these tears of sadness there is a toxic chemical that cannot be released from our bodies in any other way.[2] We can't sweat it out, pee it out, or throw it up. Just as our stomachs know how get rid of food that we can't digest, our bodies know how to release sadness in tears that spring from our eyes. Rather than trying to shut down your child's cries, reconsider encouraging him to "get all your tears out." Although crying doesn't feel good when we are doing it (just as throwing up feels awful at the time), there is a great feeling of relief after we have truly gotten all our tears out.
- *Mad* is the most destructive of our feelings and can use some emotional coaching from parents. In my experience, mad seems to be released in one of three ways, either by using one's mouth, hands, or feet.
  1. Some people release anger with their mouths: they yell, scream, bite, spit, clench, or grind their teeth. Those who can express anger with their mouths can be helped to put it into words, even if it's done loudly. Expressing anger by yelling is usually much less destructive than getting it out physically.
  2. Other people feel anger in their hands: they need to release it physically by slapping, punching, pounding, slamming, ripping, or throwing. If your youngster feels anger in his hands, he will most likely not be able to express it by "using his words." You can help this child learn to get his anger out by punching something that won't break or hurt his hands; couch cushions or beds offer a satisfying release (pillows don't usually offer enough resistance).
  3. Some people feel anger in their feet: they need to stomp, kick, or run. Kids who naturally get anger out through their feet can be

given empty egg cartons on which to stomp, a ball to kick, or taken for a jog around the neighborhood.

I believe it is important to get mad feelings out, as long as one doesn't hurt himself or anyone else in the process. My bottom line is, "It's okay to be mad, but not to be mean." Some people, when older and wiser, may learn ways to mentally release or transform anger internally. However, most folks, especially little children, need help to express anger directly in a safe way. Learning this while young will go a long toward having safe, trusting relationships when older. And, even though none of us likes to hear anger, it is important to listen to your children's angry feelings, even when they are angry with you. This is the only way we will know what our kids are feeling.

Over the years, I have had frustrated parents force teenagers into my office because their kids won't talk to them. As the teens sat there glaring sulkily, the parents explained their feelings of despair. Whenever their teens are mad, they just go to their rooms, slam the door, and refuse to tell their parents why they are angry. When I ask these parents how they handled their kids' anger when they were young, invariably the answer is, "Well, we'd just send them to their room until they got over it." Parents should be careful how they teach their toddlers to deal with angry feelings if they want their children to safely communicate those feelings to them and others when they are older. When youngsters are taught to go to their rooms and not to talk about what is bothering them, it is much harder to change that behavior later.

- *Scared* children need comfort, reassurance, and encouragement to let them know they will be kept safe and that their scared feelings will most likely "heal." It really helps to tell your children that when you were little, some things were scary for you, too, but those things were less scary as you got older. Toddlers feel great relief in knowing that they probably won't always feel so frightened. Here are a couple of helpful tips:
    1. Try to remember how frightening some things felt when you were young; this will help you not to dismiss your children's fears.

2. When helping reassure children who are scared, it is important not to either exaggerate or belittle their fears or always just rescue them. **For example:** If your child is scared of heights and becomes terrified halfway up a ladder, it would not be helpful to tell her in a panicky voice that you once knew someone who had cracked their skull from falling that distance. Nor would it help to discount her fears by exclaiming that she is just acting silly to be so scared of falling from a ladder. Either of these responses could keep her from telling you about any future fears. Climbing up the ladder and carrying her down wouldn't help her learn how to navigate such a situation in the future. What would be most helpful is saying something like, "I know you're scared, and I'll hold the ladder steady while you slowly take one step down at a time. You're doing great, each step is getting you closer and closer to the ground."

Validating a child's fearful feelings, offering reassurance, and slowly helping her problem-solve or move herself away from the frightening situation is what helps her learn to trust that you can be counted on for support when she's afraid. Children don't analyze their emotions, they just feel and express them, so it's usually not helpful at all to ask children *why* they are feeling or acting a certain way. Much better is to just validate the feelings you observe and the reasons behind those feelings, such as their difficulties with such things as waiting, sharing, or not getting something they really want. "Isn't it hard when we can't have everything we want?

---

### How a parent can help scared feelings heal by empathizing

Devon is very scared of bugs. His dad says, "I know those bugs are really scaring you." He adds, "I wonder if those bugs are scared of us, since we're so much bigger." He then shares, "I remember being scared of bugs, too, when I was a little boy, but one day they didn't seem so scary anymore. I bet that will happen for you also."

---

Makes me mad sometimes, too!" Validating your children's feelings and teaching them it's okay to "get those feelings out" will go a long way in helping your kids feel accepted and understood.

In some cultures, parents delight in the way children express feelings so openly.

When our six-month South Pacific travel adventures was drawing to a close in the Fijian Islands, Shane, then four years old, was overheard saying, "I don't want to go home. I want to stay here where they love kids." A confused looking Fijian mother questioned me, "Don't people in America love kids?" I explained that of course Americans love kids, but they tend not to enjoy childlike behavior, instead preferring children to act more like adults. The surprised mother told me that in her country adults watch the children to remind themselves how to be more playful and joyful. Fijians delight in the lively energy of children so much that it is even an honor to have a child at your dining table. If an older couple is eating alone in a restaurant, it is considered an act of kindness to send your child to eat at their table. After returning home from Fiji, it was very hard to explain to Shane why in an American restaurant, he couldn't just get up and go join any "lonely" couple he saw at another table.

Validating children's feelings helps them tune in to what they are feeling; it also makes them more self-aware, have lower stress levels, experience fewer behavioral problems, enjoy easier interpersonal relationships, and be more empathetic to others. Be prepared, however, that once you start validating your children's feelings, they may use that same strategy on you. One morning when Shane was about five years old, I was upset that my husband had taken the car that morning and had left the van for me to drive. As I complained about how I hated driving that van, Shane gently touched me on the shoulder and said, "It's okay, Mommy—I know sharing is really hard sometimes."

## Best and Worst Responses to Children's Emotions

In day-to-day dealings with your children, Mindful Parenting encourages phasing out any rejecting responses you may have heard as a child and trying to create more accepting responses instead. Consider, even as an adult, how you want others to respond to your feelings. When your feelings are validated, doesn't it help you feel understood and accepted? Validation and acceptance of children's feelings also helps them feel safe, listened to, and understood.[3]

| Feeling | Sounds of Rejection | Sounds of Acceptance |
|---|---|---|
| *Mad* | Don't talk to me that way! Get that look off your face! You are being such a bad kid! I don't want to hear about it! Go to your room until you can have a smile on your face. | Whoa, you look really mad! Looks like you've had a hard day. It's OK to be mad, but it's not OK to hurt anyone. Looks like you need to get your mad out. Here is a good way to get your mad out . . . |
| *Sad* | There's no need to cry! Big boys don't cry like that! Turn off those tears this minute! Don't be so sensitive! If you want something to cry about, I'll give you something to cry about! | Sure looks like you're feeling sad. Everyone needs to cry sometimes. Crying is a good way to get your sad out. It's good you're getting your tears out. You'll feel much better after you get all your tears out. |
| *Scared* | There's nothing to be afraid of! It's not that scary! You're acting ridiculous! You're such a sissy! Those things aren't real! Grow up! | Aren't things scary sometimes? I remember being scared of things like that when I was little. I'll help you scare them away! One day you'll probably not feel so scared by that. |
| *All Feelings (Behavior can be unacceptable, but not feelings!)* | You shouldn't feel that way. You're acting so silly! That's unacceptable! | Isn't life hard sometimes! I feel that way too sometimes. Isn't it hard to: wait, share, not get what you want, etc.? Is there anything I can do to help? Sure looks like you could use a hug. |

### Validating Any Feeling Helps

One sunny spring day, I decided to take Shane, then three years old, to the park for a picnic. We drove to the local bagel shop and bought some of our favorite foods . After I had strapped Shane back into his car seat, he began fussing and yelled loudly about wanting the food "NOW!" I was getting frustrated and, feeling that our picnic was ruined, I nearly drove back home. Then, I remembered to use my own advice about validating feeling, and said, "Isn't waiting hard? I have trouble waiting sometimes, too, especially when I'm hungry." Shane looked at me through his tears, appeared quite relieved that I understood, and immediately stopped crying. We then drove peacefully to the park and actually had a great time.

## Time-In rather than Time-Out

Helping children express their feelings is important, and no form of discipline should ever be used just because children are crying or angry, as long as they are getting their feelings out in a way that does not hurt themselves or anyone else. Discipline should be used only if children's actions are out of control, aggressive, or non-compliant (blatantly refusing to do what is asked). Remember, *punishment* means to cause pain, loss, or suffering, while *discipline* means to educate by helping one develop self-control, character, and orderly conduct.

So, here's what most parents consider the hardest part! *How can parents set clear limits on unacceptable behavior and discipline toddlers so they learn self-control without harming their children or their relationships with their kids?*

Most important is for parents to avoid any painful punishments, such as spanking (in the peaceful cultures, hitting a child would never even be considered), using consequences that are unrelated to the behavior, or enforcing Time-Outs that feel rejecting. Many parents resort to removing privileges, objects, or activities, which bring their children pleasure, that are completely unrelated to the inappropriate behavior. (Example: "Since you hit your brother, I won't let you play with your Legos today.") This type of punishment imposes a penalty that isn't logical so seems unfair to the child, doesn't require the child to change his behavior, and usually results in much resistance and resentment. Just imagine how hard it would be for any of us to regulate our emotions (calm down) if someone took away those very objects or activities that help us calm down. The goal of Mindful Parenting is not to cause suffering, but to educate children about what behavior is expected and teach them that they have the ability to change their behavior and gain your approval.

Securely-attached toddlers want their parents' approval and are usually eager to learn what behavior pleases them. Once toddlers begin to develop self-control, they won't need constant monitoring. An inner conscience emerges, just like good ole Jiminy Cricket, that reminds children what behavior is expected, even when they are away from their parents, such as being at preschool or grandma's house. This ability to self-monitor is a huge developmental leap that makes the job of parenting far easier and more enjoyable.

While I loved being a mom to my firstborn during all those early nurturing months of infancy, I dreaded the so-called "terrible twos." I knew from painful memories of my own childhood that I was unwilling to physically harm my children. So, I believed I would resort to the use of "Time-Outs," which by the mid-seventies had become a widely accepted parental alternative to physical punishment. Quite unexpectedly, however, I luckily stumbled upon a far superior method of discipline, which I realized years later when visiting Bali is similar to their method of helping kids "listen inside" in order to behave appropriately.

When my son, Shane, was fourteen months old, he began to assert his will, especially whenever I was trying to get him dressed. The two of us would struggle—as I tried to get his arm into a sleeve, he was equally determined to pull it out again. Finally, one day, at a point of utter exasperation, I sat Shane firmly on the bed and stated in an unyielding voice, "You need to stay right there until you are ready to let me get you dressed!" Then I stood back and wondered what in the heck I was doing. I had just told a baby that he needed to inform me when he was willing to cooperate, something I thought he could not yet even comprehend. Moreover, I had essentially put him in charge of when we would be able to leave the house. Knowing that we were supposed to be somewhere very soon, I anxiously pondered how I could get myself out of this embarrassing stalemate without becoming a wishy-washy parent who didn't follow through with her first attempt at limit setting. However, after just a few moments, and to my total amazement, I heard Shane's little voice say, "ready"—a word I hadn't even known he knew or understood. Then he proceeded to sit still and cooperate with getting completely dressed and out of the house in record time.

While still in shock, I realized I was on to something good! After my first trip to Bali, I chose to call this type of discipline *Time-In*, because it exemplified the Balinese belief that all children have a desire to be cooperative and can be encouraged to make the right choices when parents help them "listen-inside" to the kind of person they want to be. I experimented with this technique of "time to listen inside until you are ready to change your behavior" and used it for non-compliant behavior with both of my children. During the following thirty-five years, I have taught countless parents to successfully use Time-In with their children. Most parents are as shocked as I was to find a method of discipline that is so easy to use and rapidly helps toddlers learn to change their behavior and develop self-control.

I have found Time-In to be far superior to Time-Out because Time-Ins help a child learn that he, himself, can and must change his behavior. *Time-Ins keep the focus of behavioral change inside the child, while with Time-Outs there is external control by someone else determining how long the penalty will last, and the child may never even be required to change his behavior, which is how one develops self-control.*

During Time-Ins, the child determines how long it takes to be "ready" to do what has been asked of him; and since he is in charge of how long this takes, there is usually less resistance or resentment toward parents. Some parents question whether Time-Ins gives a child too much control. Well, the child is the only one who can *change* his behavior, but you, the parent, have complete control of what he does *until* he changes his behavior.

Another major difference is that with Time-In, a child is never sent into another room. The parent always stays with him, not holding him in an affectionate way, but just waiting; never chastising, but calmly inquiring whether he is ready to do as was asked. We want the child to realize that we don't like his behavior, and believe that he can behave appropriately. With Time-Outs when a child is sent to or locked in another room screaming, much hurt can come from feeling isolated or rejected by the parent (especially if there is a younger baby or other abandonment issues). At the other extreme is the problem of a child going to his room and just playing until being told he can come out again. In either case, the child may lack any awareness that he is expected to change his behavior, rather than just paying a penalty. Acquiring a conscience and learning how to behave in a socially appropriate manner ultimately must be developed within the child.

Remember the "balloon" example from Chapter 1 in which the Balinese mother helped her son listen inside to how he wanted to behave? The Balinese seem to maintain kindness toward their children, even when they are misbehaving, and the kids don't seem to exhibit much resistance to parental discipline.

Time-Ins are used to help a child "listen inside" to develop self control and can be initiated as soon as a toddler begins to understand cause and effect, which happens sometime between the ages of fourteen and eighteen months. You will sense the time is right when you notice that gleam of awareness in your toddler's eye as you tell her not to throw her banana on the floor, and she knowingly looks right at you, grins, and does it anyway. While allowing and helping children express their feelings is important, a parent must not permit children's behavior to be blatantly disobedient. You want to teach your children that if you ask them to do something, you expect them to cooperate. It may be helpful if you attempt to playfully engage a positive response like challenging your toddler with, "I bet I can get all these dishes into the kitchen before you get that banana picked up," or use the "when and then" approach: "When you pick up that banana, then I will read you a book." However, if your toddler still refuses to do as she's told, Time-In will be your most useful tool in dealing with such deliberate lack of cooperation.

## When and How to Use Time-In

When your toddler refuses to be cooperative, such as throwing the banana on the floor, after you asked her not to do that, clearly state what you want her to do. "Please pick the banana up off of the floor." If she is still unwilling to do it, firmly tell her that she needs to sit down wherever she is (or in a previously designated "ready seat" such as a certain chair, pillow, or bottom step of the stairway) until she is "ready" to pick up the banana. Then, just calmly wait with her until she is ready. You may ask, "Are you ready to pick up the banana now?" If she isn't ready, then tell her to stay seated until she *is* ready. As soon as the child says or indicates that she is ready, even if she is angry or crying, she is immediately invited to get up, pick up the banana, and then do whatever she pleases. Occasionally, your child may test you by saying she is ready, but then doesn't follow through. Try to remain calm, and respond with, "Whoops, you made a mistake. You thought you were ready, but you aren't quite ready yet. Go back and sit down until you are *really* ready." This approach should initially only be used when there is enough time to allow the child to become "ready,"

### Time-In Leads to Self-Control

A few years ago, two worried parents came to my office concerned about their son's aggressive behavior toward the family dog. Kevin was four years old and had become quite aggressive and non-compliant. Kevin's parents were overly permissive and had great difficulty with limit setting. I explained the Time-In method and suggested that Kevin really needed to learn self-control, and as parents, they needed to be firm in making sure he sat in Time-In until he really was ready to act appropriately. Kevin's reluctant parents did not believe that Time-In would work. I convinced them to just try it consistently for two weeks. After ten days, I received a call from Kevin's mother. She excitedly explained that she had just walked past the living room and saw Kevin sitting on the "ready seat." When she asked him why he was sitting there, Kevin said, "I was going to hit the dog, and I'm sitting here until I'm ready to stop doing that."

not when you need to race out the door. However, with consistent use it usually doesn't take more than a couple of weeks for a child to start becoming "ready" fairly quickly and the need to sit in the "ready seat" greatly decreases.

In the unusual case that your child refuses to stay seated, you may need to hold her until she is ready. While holding her, perhaps on your lap facing away from you, make sure that she can't hit (holding her arms down if necessary), kick, or slam into you with her head. Be certain that you are not holding her in a nurturing way that could reinforce her misbehavior. Remember, the bottom line while disciplining is to not let anyone get hurt, including you. If this type of discipline is initiated with an older child after years of using externally controlling or exceedingly permissive methods, it may take a little longer before the child clearly understands, accepts, and learns that she can and must change her behavior.

So, how about parenting children with whom you do not have a secure attachment due to a difficult beginning, or with foster, adopted, or stepchildren? Time-In is still the recommended method of discipline, although it may take awhile before parents see a positive change in the children's self-monitoring of behaviors. Children hurt by the lack of a close relationship during their first year of life have great difficulty trusting others, so need even more kindness, patience, and consistency to open their hearts to a new relationship. The importance of feeling safe in order to develop trust makes it a necessity for punishing parenting practices to never be

## Time-Ins Create Safety

One nine-year-old client of mine who had grown up in foster care often became out of control during the first year that I worked with her. I had to hold her quite a few times until she was "ready" to stop trying to hurt herself or me. Even now, thirty years later, she sometimes contacts me. She recently said, "You were the only person I ever really trusted to keep me safe and not hurt me. I think the reason I now am so good with kids and do my best to make others happy is because you helped me realize I was a good person inside."

used, as they could further damage such children's ability to trust adults. I believe that all children have a core of goodness inside that can be tapped into by someone who is fair and kind. (Even antisocial personality disorder, which may have a genetic basis, is believed to be triggered by family relations and environmental factors.) The younger children are, the easier it is for them to develop trusting relationships. Such trust must be built before unattached children will want to cooperate. Start building trust by first validating their feelings, which will help them feel understood, then clearly let them know your expectations, and follow this with suggestions of ways they can cooperate. Time-In should *only be used for unsafe behavior or blatant non-compliance*. Attachment-challenged children will usually experience Time-In as fair and non-threatening. Time-Out on the other hand can retrigger feelings of rejection and abandonment, while corporal punishment, or removal of comfort objects or activities can reinforce the belief that adults are uncaring and should not be trusted.

Some well-meaning parents are ill advised to use forceful holding as a way to coerce unattached children to make eye contact attempting to encourage an attachment. I can't imagine that such treatment would ever help me fall in love with someone, can you? While physically holding may be necessary for children who are out of control or not willing to stay in a Time-In situation, it should only be used until the child is under control or "ready" to engage in the expected behavior and never be attempted as a method of relationship building.

We all know that parents are more willing to readily use a form of discipline when it doesn't create lots of anger and screaming from either the parent or the child. One of the great benefits of Time-In is that parents tend to use it quickly, as soon as there is non-compliance, rather than making several requests and giving repeated warnings until they finally become angry themselves. Anytime parents lack control of their own anger, there is the potential to be harmful to their children, no matter what form of punishment or discipline they attempt to use. The only situation in which I recommend the use of Time-Out is for overwhelmed parents to remove themselves from the situation in order to take a break, calm down, and reconsider how they can best help their children learn the desired behavior.

The expectation that all kids want to be cooperative and have positive loving connections can lead to healthier relationships within families. In Bali a special intervention is held if an older Balinese child or adult has done something that was especially painful to someone in the family. This cleansing ceremony is a way to express pain toward the family member who has hurt others and allow for healing of those relationships. It is held at a local temple and conducted by the village priest with all concerned members of the extended family present. I was once permitted to watch such an intimate family event. After the priest blessed the family and offerings were placed around the temple, a school-aged boy was brought up to the front. While his grandfather offered him support, his father, mother, uncle, and grandmother each were given a chance to express their anger and sadness. I never understood what the boy had done wrong, but it was amazing to watch such an incredible family catharsis, resulting in the boy showing his regret and then reconnecting in a positive open-hearted way with each member of the family. The ability to release painful feelings and allow for personal accountability, along with expectations of forgiveness seems like such a beneficial way of dealing with difficult family issues.

Taking personal responsibility for one's behavior and developing self-control are extremely important lessons for children to learn and have a tremendous impact on overall happiness. A recent long-term study in New Zealand of one thousand people observed from birth to age thirty-two indicated that self-control made a great difference in leading a successful life. Self-control in this research was defined as using skills such as self-discipline, considering the potential consequences of one's actions, and being reliable. When these research participants got older, self-control in some cases made the difference between getting a good job or going to jail. The researchers found that "the children who struggled with self-control as preschoolers were three times more likely to have problems as young adults. They were more prone to have a criminal record, more likely to be poor or have financial problems, and they were more likely to be single parents."[5]

Expectations of accountability and consistent use of Time-In with toddlers can help them from very early in life to develop a strong conscience along with self-control that will eliminate years of continued monitoring. Cooperative children not only make the job of parenting much more enjoyable, but such self-discipline will be a great gift to them in terms of future success in school, jobs, relationships, and overall happiness throughout the rest of their lives.

# CHAPTER 6

# Brain Development:
# The Power of Nurturing

*Only the proper environmental conditions are required to allow the*
*underlying and natural "seed of compassion" to germinate and grow.*
—Dalai Lama

In the past ten years, there has been an unbelievable explosion in knowledge concerning early brain development. Assumptions that psychologists have long made about the way events very early in childhood influence later personality, relationships, and overall success in life are now being validated. The Tibetans have apparently known for thousands of years that parents have a direct impact on their developing baby while in utero. This information has provided pregnant couples with suggestions during each week of gestation regarding how they can support the healthy physical and emotional development of their unborn offspring. Western brain researchers are now finding that environmental factors during pregnancy, birth, and a baby's first few years have tremendous lifelong effects on such abilities as: self-calming, creative problem-solving, self-esteem, self-control, trust, compassion, and empathy.

## Blending Ancient Wisdom with Modern Science

All human infants in the world are born having the same biological and emotional needs. It is believed that the way children are raised helps them better adapt to the culture in which they live. While this may be true for toddlers and older children, the basic physical and emotional needs of infants are universally the same, regardless of the culture into which they are born.

How can we help infants get the best possible start so that they reach their highest potentials? Attempts are being made across many scientific fields, including anthropology, psychology, and neuroscience, to determine exactly which parenting practices promote the most positive infant development. Anthropologist Meredith Small uses the term "ethnopediatrics" to describe the evolutionary, cross-cultural, and biological factors of parenting that are most desirable for human infants.[1]

Although no culture has all the answers to something as complex as parenting, we live in a technological age where information can be gathered and easily shared among nearly every culture in the world. The ability now exists to discover which parenting practices are best for the healthy development of babies' bodies and brains. Even though our lifestyles may be different from people living in small rural villages of developing countries, if their caregiving practices are better at meeting infants' needs, shouldn't we try to implement them? Blending some of the best worldwide parenting wisdom with findings from cutting edge brain research could prove incredibly valuable in helping raise future generations of healthier, happier, and more peaceful people.

## Prenatal Brain Development

At the Institute of HeartMath, Doc Childre and his colleagues have learned that forty to sixty percent of our heart cells are brain (neural) cells connected to the emotional (limbic) part of our brains.[2] Since the heart is the first organ to begin functioning in the developing fetus, it is now assumed that emotional information is being recorded there throughout most of the pregnancy. Knowledge as to whether a baby is safe and wanted, along with information concerning the environment outside the womb, is received by the fetus from the mother's perceptions of life, including her feelings of contentment, happiness, sadness, anger, stress, and fear.

As a psychologist, I have found that people who were adopted into a loving adoptive home, even if immediately after birth, often have deep feelings of rejection, angst, and anxiety about being loveable. Knowing that emotional information is recorded during gestation helps us understand how this could occur for a fetus growing in the womb of a woman faced with the painful realization that she might not be able to keep her baby.

If we stop to think about our own strong emotions, we realize that love and deep emotional pain are definitely felt in our hearts rather than in our heads. When someone feels loving, she experiences herself as "open-hearted." A common response to feeling betrayed is "my heart aches" or "I'm broken-hearted." If deeply hurt, we sense our "hearts close down." When making important emotional decisions, aren't we constantly reminded to "follow our hearts?" We even use a heart-shaped symbol to represent expressions of love. There is a growing acceptance that the heart is more than just an organ which pumps blood throughout our bodies. It is being understood as central to guiding our emotional lives by sending signals to the body and brain that help them work together in harmony.

Historically, it has been believed that the genes a baby inherits during conception control the development of his body and mind, and that all a pregnant woman needed to do was eat well and wait nine months for the baby to emerge. But current research shows that a pregnant mother has a great deal of influence over who her baby will become, because the environment a mother creates in her womb has tremendous influence on the developing fetus. While this is exciting news, it can also create a great deal of anxiety for gestating mothers, who are unsure of what they should or should not be doing to best benefit their unborn babies. Some people believe that letting a woman know how much influence she has over her developing fetus may cause too much fear and guilt. While no one should be blamed for previously being unaware of the potential impact mothers have on their developing offspring, now that we know such consequences exist, this knowledge ought to be shared. Parents deserve as much information as possible concerning what is likely to influence the development of their unborn baby, even though no mother can control everything that happens in her life in order to have a "perfect" pregnancy.

Thomas Verny, MD, a Canadian leader in the field of prenatal and perinatal psychiatry, states in his book *Pre-Parenting*, "From the moment of conception, the experience in the womb shapes the brain and lays the groundwork for personality, emotional temperament, and the power of higher thought."[3] Bernie Devlin, a professor of psychiatry, has found that "fifty-one percent of a child's potential intelligence is controlled by environmental factors."[4] This includes negative factors in utero such as decreased blood flow to the fetus when a pregnant mother drinks alcohol or smokes cigarettes.

A fetus is influenced not only by what is happening in the environment outside the womb, but also how the mother perceives and deals with that environment. Stress hormones cross the placenta, so the mother's emotional state during pregnancy directly affects the developing brain of her baby. Even when stressful events occur, a pregnant woman who has nurturing support from family and friends along with methods of stress relief can help create a more positive internal environment in which her unborn baby is growing. In 2011, a BBC News article entitled "Mum's stress is passed to baby in the womb" explained that continued high-level stress, throughout a pregnancy, as opposed to common everyday minor stresses, is what leads to long-term ill effects.[5]

Bruce Lipton, PhD, an internationally recognized cell biologist, explains in *The Biology of Belief* that the actual genes of a developing baby are selected in response to the environment experienced in the womb. In utero, the baby's brain develops from the primitive hindbrain that controls survival to the higher-functioning cerebral cortex.

In a very stressful pregnancy, hormones direct the fetal blood to nourish the baby's arms, legs, and hindbrain to increase the infant's chances of survival after birth, while suppressing the development of the forebrain where intelligence, problem solving, and creativity reside. It makes sense that if a baby is being born into an especially dangerous environment, the flight-fight protective skills would be more crucial to survival than advanced levels of reasoning. On the other hand, a mother who feels

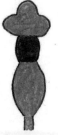 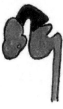 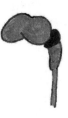 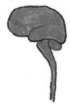

20 days          6 weeks          12 weeks          24 weeks

relatively calm and secure during pregnancy helps her baby develop an enlarged forebrain and a smaller hindbrain.[6]

In Dr. Lipton's workshops, he often presents an unforgettable video of a fetal ultrasound. It was made by the Italian conscious-parenting organization, Associazione Nazionale per l'Educazione Prenatale, and shows a fetus floating peacefully in the womb until his parents get into a loud argument. When the fighting begins, the fetus immediately startles, and the baby's body arches as the yelling increases. At the sound of shattering glass, the fetus literally jumps several inches high. To anyone watching this video, there is no doubt that the external environment, along with the adrenaline pumping through the mother's body, directly affected that baby in utero.

## Brain Development After Birth

Have you ever wondered why our babies are born so helpless? Why other newborn mammals can feed themselves very soon after birth, but it takes a human infant nine more months to be able to do that? It appears that humans are born nine months prematurely because of the size of their brains. When our primitive ancestors began to stand upright, their pelvic girdles got smaller to allow them to balance and more easily walk on two legs. This also freed up the use of their hands, which could be used for a multitude of new tasks. As early humans creatively began using their hands, their brains started to enlarge, thus making it necessary for their babies to be born much earlier to fit through the birth canal.

Today, human infants appear to be born only halfway through their gestation, resulting in most of their brain-growth taking place after birth. And although human newborns are totally and utterly helpless, at least their primitive hindbrain has developed sufficiently enough by the time they are born to allow them to cry out for help. Newborns who are moved even three feet away from their mothers scream loudly in terror because they are completely defenseless and only feel secure when they can see, feel, or smell the only familiar haven of safety that they have ever known. It is critical for their mothers or other nurturing caregivers to answer infants' distressed cries, which reduces their feelings of panic and helps

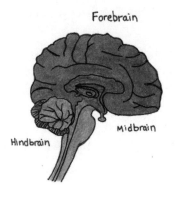

Forebrain

Midbrain

Hindbrain

begin development of trust that they will be protected during the next nine months as they complete their gestational development. When infants' and toddlers' cries are responded to as soon as possible, there is a decrease in stress hormones, allowing stimulation to move toward developing the higher functioning social and emotional parts of the brain.

The cortex is the forebrain's outer layer of neural tissue. The greatest growth of an infant's prefrontal cortex takes place from *six to nine months after birth*, making this an especially important time for the baby to continue receiving lots of attention and nurturing from an attached, responsive caregiver. Stanley Greenspan, MD, known for his

## Brain Development
## (From the Brainstem Upward)

### Forebrain:

- Cortex—Reasoning, Logic, Awareness, Consciousness, Regulating emotions
- Socialization, Compassion, Empathy
- Cerebrum—Thoughts, Speech, Judgment, Motor activity, Sensory perceptions, Working memory

### Midbrain:

- Limbic System—Emotions and Long-term memory
- Pituitary Gland—Hormone regulation

### Hindbrain:

- Cerebellum—Motor activities, Balance, Coordination
- Brainstem—Survival

research on the way basic structures in human brains are developed from interactions between infants and their devoted caregivers, states that "Consistent, nurturing relationships with the same caregivers early in life are the cornerstones of emotional and intellectual competence."[7] These findings are echoed by Alan Shore, PhD, professor in the Department of Psychiatry at the UCLA School of Medicine, who has found that the ability of a child to regulate emotions is greatly enhanced by secure, responsive, and sensitive relationships.[8] It is unfortunate that most six- to nine-month-old American babies currently are not spending much of their day with a loving parent during this critical stage of prefrontal brain development.

Why is the prefrontal cortex so important? This is the part of the brain that is referred to as the "civilized brain." It is responsible for increased intelligence, creativity, regulation of emotions (self-calming), reading, responding to social cues, problem solving, judging long-term consequences, and for the capability to be compassionate, empathetic, and loving. I have noticed that many toddlers in peaceful cultures have very large protruding foreheads. Could this be due, as some believe, to the growth of larger prefrontal lobes? (See photo 18.)

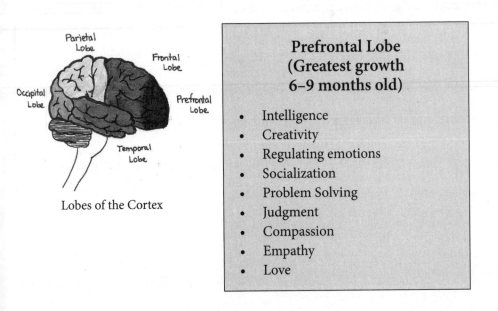

Lobes of the Cortex

**Prefrontal Lobe
(Greatest growth
6–9 months old)**

- Intelligence
- Creativity
- Regulating emotions
- Socialization
- Problem Solving
- Judgment
- Compassion
- Empathy
- Love

In Sue Gerhardt's noteworthy book, *Why Love Matters: How Affection Shapes a Baby's Brain,* she explains that the prefrontal part of the brain helps us restrain from acting out feelings of rage. It serves to calm our fears, while increasing our self-control, will power, and the ability to empathize with others by "experiencing" what they are feeling.[9] These particularly important qualities are essential if we are attempting to grow kinder children who are able to resolve conflicts instead of becoming bullies who merely resort to hindbrain fight-flight mechanisms of protection. Empathy is critical if we want to create a world that is less violent, more compassionate, and ultimately peaceful.

The rate of brain growth in the first few years of babies' lives makes their brains much more vulnerable to damage than adults' brains. Since babies' brains are underdeveloped, with neurons still rapidly creating connections (synapses), the brains of neglected infants become structurally different than those of nurtured infants. Stress causes increased levels of cortisol, an adrenal hormone that has been found to be neurotoxic, causing harm to brain cells and sometimes even killing them. Lowering stress in babies is essential for building a healthy brain, and this can be done most quickly by holding, carrying, rocking, singing, gently stroking, or massaging a baby. All kinds of tender touches are exceptionally calming to infants. Balinese babies are never out of someone's arms for the first three months of life, and the Tibetans believe that touch is extremely important for healthy brain development. Never be afraid to pick up your crying baby and give her as much attention as she desires, because this will help her become an emotionally healthy and loving child.

A recent study with rats showed how and why being touched is so essential to a developing brain. In a *Psychology Today* article, Alex Korb, PhD, reported that baby rats, which were nurtured by mothers that spent considerable time licking them, showed less fear, had lowered stress hormones, and were more resilient in stressful situations than baby rats that were not licked as much. Apparently, there are two types of rat mothers; those that are high-level lickers and those that are low-level lickers. Being licked releases the good love hormone, oxytocin, that promotes feelings of connection and reduces stress. When female baby rats of "high-licking" mothers later became mothers themselves, they also did a lot of licking of their babies. Baby female rats of the "low-licking" mothers grew up to be much more anxious and became "low-licking" mothers with their own babies. To determine whether the anxiety level was genetic, some of the infant rats were switched from their "low-licking" mothers and placed with "high-licking" moms. The babies adopted by "high-licking" mothers ended up with lower stress and anxiety than their siblings that had remained with their "low-licking" mothers. These results indicate that with regard to anxiety in baby rats, environmental factors play a more crucial role than genetics. The amount of nurturing received seems to govern the baby rats' stress levels and overall degree of contentment in their lives.[10]

James W. Prescott, PhD, a developmental neuropsychologist and former director of the National Institute of Child Health and Human Development, has studied the lifelong impact of early mother-infant nurturing on the developing brain of primates. In his experiments with newborn monkeys, he found that sensory stimulation through intimate touch and affection was essential for normal brain development both structurally and functionally. Dr. Prescott's research repeatedly concluded that the failure of mother-infant attachment led to brain abnormalities and biochemical deficiency that brought about anxiety, depression, alienation, anger, rage, and violence.[11]

In a human study, Mary Carlson, a neurobiologist at Harvard Medical School, studied anxiety in Romanian orphans who ranged in age from a few months to three years old by measuring their saliva cortisol levels. She determined that lack of touching and attention, along with poor-quality day care led to higher cortisol levels that stunted the children's growth and had a negative effect on their behavior. The higher the stress, the poorer was the outcome for the child.[12]

Although it was historically believed in the US that babies who were held *too much* or given *lots of* attention would become spoiled, overly dependent, or otherwise damaged, current brain research and observations of babies in cultures with extensive nurturing is proving that idea to be completely false. It appears that no matter what genes babies inherit, it is parenting and environmental factors that determine whether children become aggressive or compassionate. The current rate of childhood emotional distress and the large number of medications prescribed for young American children with mental health issues could be the result of generations of children being raised by parents who did not give *enough attention* to their infants.

Now provided with the knowledge that babies thrive on attention, touch, and nurturing for optimal brain development, blending parenting practices from peaceful cultures along with findings from early brain research can hopefully transform the parenting of our babies. By giving infants as much attention and physical affection as possible, especially during the first year of life, we can begin promoting development of brain structures that can promisingly lead to greater lifelong mental and emotional health.

## Promoting Compassion and Empathy

With today's increased incidences of childhood bullying and far too many horrendous school shootings in which teens are killing not only each other, but even very young children, it is especially crucial to investigate what, exactly, promotes compassion and empathy. Compassion is care, kindness, and concern for another, while empathy is the ability to feel something from another person's point of view.

A baby is born with seeds of empathy accompanying their built-in ability and immediate need to form a close intimate relationship with a parent or nurturing caregiver. The infant's basic survival depends on developing a mutual relationship with a mother, father, or another caring adult who can empathize enough with her that she knows all her needs will be understood and met. When she is hungry—she will be fed; when air becomes trapped in her belly—she will be burped; when cold— warmed; when wet—changed; when sad or scared—comforted; when bored—given attention; when lonely—held, caressed, and reassured. Being treated with consistent attempts to alleviate her discomfort by an empathetic caregiver reduces an infant's stress by helping her feel understood, comforted, and safe. It also helps her begin to build mental connections between having needs and being able to trust another person to provide sensitive, caring relief. These connections provide the necessary foundation for a child's ability to believe that relationships are desirable, enable her to feel worthy of being loved, and help grow her ability to experience trust, empathy, and love toward others.

Humans thrive when they can form close *interdependent* relationships. They have never survived well independently, always needing the protection of cooperative groups. Historically, clans were formed in which people worked together to gather food, build shelter, care for the children, and protect each other from predators. American parents often talk of wanting their children to be independent; however the ability to be *inter*dependent is actually the greatest gift we can give our children. I think fondly of how lucky the Balinese children are to live in extended-family compounds with the overwhelming amount of attention and love they get. There are at least four loving adults constantly watching, playing, and adoring each child in the family. Helping children develop social skills and learn to live cooperatively leads them to having closer lifelong relationships with their family members, friends, partners, and eventually their own children.

Neurocience journalist Maia Szalavitz and child psychiatrist Bruce Perry, MD, PhD, in their recently published book *Born For Love: Why Empathy is Essential—and Endangered,* write, "Empathy underlies virtually everything that makes society work—like trust, altruism, collaboration, love, [and] charity. Failure to empathize is a key part of most social problems—crime, violence, war, racism, child abuse, and inequity . . . ."[13] If parents make a conscious effort to cultivate empathy in their children our society will be transformed. I am convinced that the reason the Tibetans, Bhutanese, and Balinese have peaceful cultures is that they make such an effort to nurture this quality in their children. When I asked Dr. Mimi Lhamu, a pediatrician in Bhutan, what is the most important thing a parent can do to raise a compassionate child, she gave me a puzzled "isn't that obvious" look and then answered quickly, "Well, you must treat them with compassion."[14]

## Parenting for Optimal Brain Development

In past generations, there was a commonly held belief that anything that happened to children before they could talk (at about age three) really didn't matter, because they would have no memory of it. We now know that early experiences, which begin in utero, essentially shape a child's brain, and those that occur before age three have the greatest impact on a child's social and emotional development.

This knowledge can be both exciting and terrifying. Never before have Westerners realized that very early parenting has such tremendous impact in forming a child into the person he becomes. My Balinese friends believe that a parent's job is to help a child become the best at whomever he is truly meant to be, but that a parent should never try to control, manipulate, or change who that child is to become. As an avid gardener, I understand what this means. If I have a young cherry tree, I won't try to make it grow plums. But if I nurture and care for the tree well, I can help it become a healthy tree with strong branches, lush green leaves, and delicious sweet cherries.

This is also true for growing beautiful, self-actualized children. The mindful attention and encouragement that infants and toddlers receive from their parents create connections between different parts of the baby's brain. Neuropsychiatrist Daniel Siegel, MD, in his book *The Whole Brain Child*, explains that when parents spend time interacting with their youngsters, it helps to integrate the different parts of their children's brains, which leads to "improved decision making, better control of body and emotions, fuller self-understanding, stronger relationships, and success in school."[15]

Knowing when specific parts of a child's brain are developing can help parents become aware of what an infant or toddler needs at that particular stage. However, what is most important for parents to remember during the first eighteen months of an infant's life is to form a close, secure attachment and take delight in caring for, holding, touching, playing with, listening and responding to, and keeping that baby as close as possible throughout the day and nighttime. When parents enjoy being with their infant (even though none of us like being awoken during the night) and can cherish those sweet smiles and soft coos, then there is nothing to worry about. If the relationship is pleasing to both the parent and infant, the baby's prefrontal lobe will develop in an optimum fashion.

Stranger anxiety and separation anxiety that emerge separately some-time between six and twelve months of age are healthy signs of a secure attachment and normal social brain development. When a closely attached parent is out of sight, an infant cannot understand that the cherished parent still exists. Repeated separations and long periods of being away from a dearly loved attachment figure can adversely affect a baby's developing brain because of increased levels of damaging cortisol that accompany the fear of losing the person on whom the baby is most dependent.

The US is one of the few countries in the world in which babies, by twelve weeks of age, are often separated from their working parents for most of the day. Sixty-one percent of children under the age of five in the US attend day care programs because their parents work outside the home. The question of whether day care is helpful or harmful to young children has been the topic of controversy for decades. Now, provided with the understanding that stress hormones are damaging to a developing brain, along with the fact that cortisol samples can be taken easily using a quick saliva sample, we are better able to settle this debate.

In 1999, American researchers Andrea Dettling and her colleagues studied the cortisol levels of toddlers who were separated from their parents for the entire day in a group childcare situation. While these youngsters' behavior did not appear stressed, their cortisol levels rose to a very high level throughout the day, especially in children with poor social skills.[16] A year later, Dettling found that toddlers kept in their homes with highly responsive nannies had normal levels of cortisol throughout the day.[17]

Dr. Megan Gunnar, a well-known researcher of childcare stress at the University of Minnesota, created an easy method of testing cortisol in which rolls of cotton dipped in flavored sugar crystals are given to babies to suck on and the saliva is then analyzed to determine stress levels. Dr. Gunnar found that when babies are cared for at home, their cortisol levels start out high in the morning, but decrease throughout the day. Gunnar found, however, that seventy to eighty percent of toddlers and preschoolers in full-time day care had cortisol levels that continued to increase throughout the day. Poor quality care, long hours, multiple caregivers, many different settings, and the younger a baby is when placed in day care all lead to increased levels of cortisol. Youngsters who were shy, fearful, or had trouble calming themselves suffered the most. The good news was that when babies had close secure attachments with highly nurturing mothers or primary caregivers for the first four to six months of life, when later placed in day care their cortisol levels tended to remain stable. Consistently, the younger the child is when placed in an out-of-home day care situation, the greater is the risk of harm to the child's development.[18]

Researchers such as Gordon Neufeld, PhD, and Gabor Maté, MD, explain in their best-seller, *Hold On to Your Kids: Why Parents Need to Matter More Than Peers,* that early separation and loss of adult attachment figures are responsible for American teens being more attached to and influenced by their peers than by their parents. Neufeld and Maté remind us that this is the first time in human history that young children are not growing up with nurturing caregivers to whom they are related. Today's kids are not attached to an extended family, clan, or neighborhood and many do not even have intact nuclear families. Lack of time spent with consistent adult relationships leads kids quite early to seek out peer mentors. This change in early care of our children has paralleled the increase in childhood bullying, violence, and suicide.[19]

Linda Lantieri, an author, educator, and administrator in New York City, who has been dedicated over the past thirty years to conflict resolution and resilience in students, reports that children's social and emotional development has seriously declined over the past few decades. Kids seem sadder and lonelier, exhibiting more aggressive, disobedient, and impulsive behaviors. Lantieri and Daniel Goleman's book *Building Emotional Intelligence* reminds us that kids today are faced with current-day stressors that did not existed previously. They cite a national Kids Poll that surveyed 875 children from the ages of nine through thirteen concerning what causes them stress and what helps them cope with it. An astonishing seventy-five percent of the kids stated that they needed their parents to spend more time with them when they were going through a difficult time.[20] (See Chapter 8 for suggestions about how countless modern parents are finding creative ways to balance financial pressures and career obligations while still meeting the relational needs of their young children.)

## Consequences of Poor Attachment

As explained in Chapter 2, there are three primary types of mother-infant attachment: secure attachment, insecure attachment, and unattached. Although typically referring to mothers, this applies to any caregivers to whom infants have their first primary attachments. Without a secure primary attachment to a caring adult in the first two years of life, a baby's prefrontal cortex does not develop in a healthy way. Some observations by Dr. Harold Chugani and his colleagues have shown that Romanian orphaned babies who were unattached to any caregiver and left alone in cribs most of the day had virtually no brain activity in their prefrontal area.[21] When this part of the brain does not develop normally in the first few years of life, there is very little chance of later recovering these lost abilities to form interpersonal relationships and engage in higher-level prefrontal brain activity.

Early attachment problems interfere with the social-emotional development of the brain, which leads to the following *long-term* consequences:

- ***Insecure Attachment:*** Difficulties exist in problem solving, regulating emotions, having healthy relationships, and trusting oneself or others.
- ***Unattached:*** Young children exhibit very contradictory responses, such as approach and then avoidant behaviors with caregivers, excessive familiarity with strangers, and resistance to comforting. Persistent lifelong personality disorders are later apparent with difficulties in interpersonal relationships, abnormal emotional responses, anger, impulse control, and significant impairment in social and occupational functioning.

Parenting is the most demanding and exhausting of all jobs, and if a parent does not feel a loving attachment to a child, it can lead to that child being neglected or abused.

When this occurs during the earliest months and years of a child's life, that child becomes hurt, lacks empathy (due to not being treated with empathy), and can become aggressive. *This is how bullies are made!* Research has shown that neglect is just as likely as abuse to lead to later

| Type of Attachment | Mother's Behavior | Baby's Behavior |
|---|---|---|
| Secure | *Nurturing and Responding quickly to baby's needs* | *Cries less* *Easily comforted* |
| Insecure | ***Unpredictable:*** *Doesn't read baby's cues* *Parenting by the clock* *Responds in a negative manner* | *Cries a great deal* *Demanding* *Anxious* *Difficult to soothe* |
| Unattached | *Disregards baby's physical and emotional needs* | *Avoids physical contact* *Resists comforting* *Unresponsive* |

criminal conduct caused by lack of respect for the rights of others. While most abuse survivors do not become violent criminals, they are at much greater risk of engaging in criminal behavior and of becoming abusive parents with their own children.

In the US, more than one thousand children a year die from abuse and neglect, and tens of thousands of kids grow up to become violent criminals. A recent study by Prevent Child Abuse America revealed that the direct and indirect costs of child neglect and abuse were found to be more than $100 billion a year. Every child who drops out of school and becomes a career criminal will cost society an average of $2.5 million over their lifetime. Fight Crime: Invest in Kids is an organization of law enforcement workers, district attorneys, and violence survivors throughout the US that works to help children get early protection from neglect and abuse. In their 2009 report, programs were described that have been highly successful in helping very young at-risk children and are estimated to save tax payers from three to five dollars for each dollar that was invested.[22] These findings confirm that it is not only easier to build a healthy child than repair a damaged adult, but it is also much less expensive.

## Early Stress Affects Mind and Body

The early stress experienced by neglected and abused children leaves marks on their minds and bodies. We usually think of such kids as resilient survivors, but we fail to notice that their long-term mental and physical health may have been significantly affected by those early experiences.

Robin Karr-Morse's recent book *Scared Sick: The Role of Childhood Trauma in Adult Disease* explains the important connection between trauma and disease and how this discovery was made.[23] The National Institute on Drug Abuse has observed that people with obesity, alcoholism, and drug addiction all have below-normal levels of dopamine in their brains. Dopamine is a pleasure hormone, and these individuals tend to get addicted to substances that create a temporary increase in dopamine. In the 1980s, at Kaiser Permanente Hospital in San Diego, California, Vincent Felitti, MD, began to focus on preventive care in family medicine rather than just on treating the symptoms of illnesses. In a clinic created for chronically obese patients, it was quickly discovered that these patients associated food with pleasure and also protection from feeling vulnerable to physical, emotional, or sexual abuse. When patients began losing weight, they would become increasingly anxious. This connection between childhood trauma and later illness began to be investigated.

Dr. Felitti and Robert Anda, MD, collaboratively developed the Adverse Childhood Experiences (ACE) Study. The ACE questionnaire focused on

## Early Traumas Leading to Later Health Problems[24]

- Gestating in a Highly Stressed Mother
- Prenatal Alcohol
- Prematurity
- Unnecessary Birth Interventions
- Maternal Depression
- Early Separations
- Painful Medical Practices
- Inadequate Childcare
- Domestic Violence
- Divorce and Custody Issues
- Death of a Parent

questions concerning emotional, physical, and sexual abuse, along with childhood experiences of growing up in a household that included: (1) alcoholism or drug abuse; (2) someone who was chronically depressed, mentally ill, or suicidal; (3) domestic violence of the mother; (4) incarceration of a household member; and (5) parents who were separated, divorced, or in any other way lost during childhood. What Drs. Felitti, Anda, and their colleagues concluded is that "early childhood trauma can lead to an array of negative health outcomes and behaviors . . . " The greater the number of early adverse experiences children have, the greater the prevalence of later risk-taking and addictive behaviors, such as overeating, risky sex, and the use of alcohol, nicotine, and other drugs. All these behaviors lead to a release of dopamine and thereby appear to be methods of self-comforting. A strong correlation has also been found between adverse childhood experiences and the risk of attempted suicide throughout the individual's life.[25]

Dr. Anda believes that stress or trauma in prenatal, infant, and toddler stages are the most significant factors leading to poor long-term health outcomes. Karr-Morse explains that if young children experience terror when they are very helpless, it leads to toxic levels of cortisol resulting in an overwhelming "freeze" response. While kids can recover from single extremely stressful events without harm, an increased number of traumas early in life can lead to chronic levels of cortisol accumulation that trigger outcomes such as inflammatory and immune dysfunctions.

In the past, it was believed that most diseases had a genetic explanation, but even this is now being questioned. While some diseases are definitely inherited, such as Sickle-Cell and Cystic Fibrosis, the ACE studies are indicating that a multitude of diseases appear to be triggered by an interaction between genetics, physiology, and prolonged negative emotions such as fear, shame, and rage that are experienced early in life.

Emotional abuse caused by bullying, which has seriously increased in our country, is also being linked to later difficulties with health, finances, jobs, relationships, and criminal felonies. Research done by William Copeland, an associate professor at Duke University School of Medicine, found that children who were targets of bullying later became adults who were much more likely to suffer from serious health problems such as

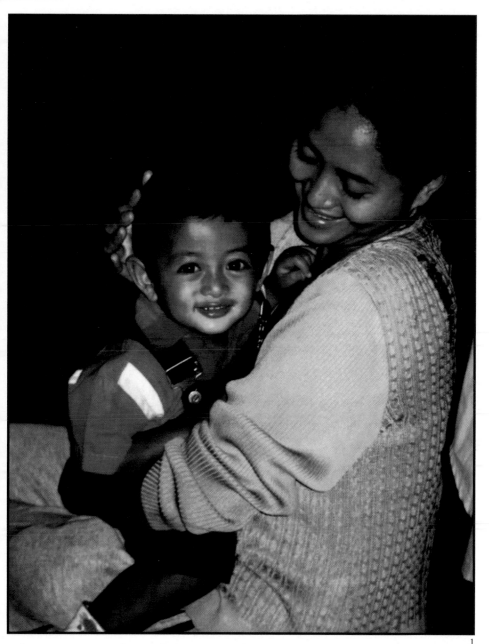

When parents respond in gentle, loving ways, they grow calm, kind, and delightful children.[1]

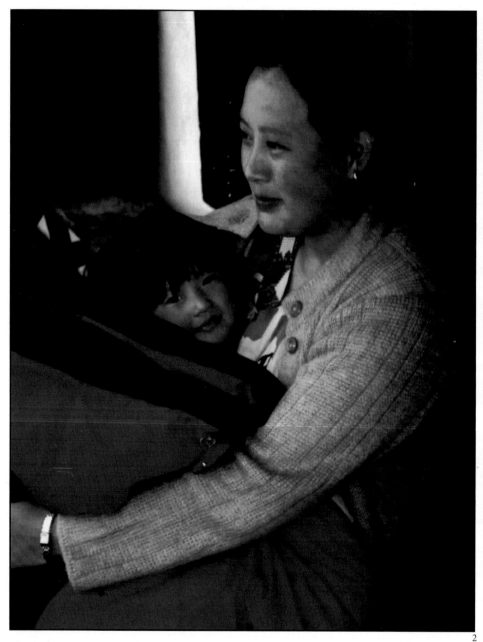

The Dalai Lama is certain that we learn how to love from our mothers, and that this first relationship sets the tone for all future relationships.

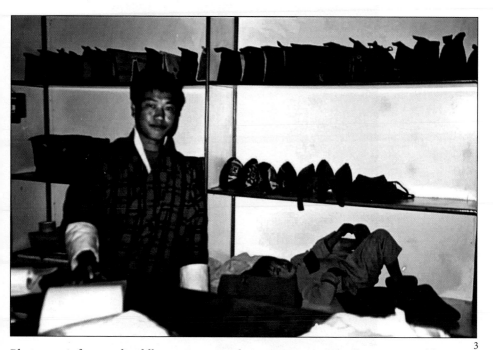

3

Bhutanese infants and toddlers accompany their parents to work whenever possible.

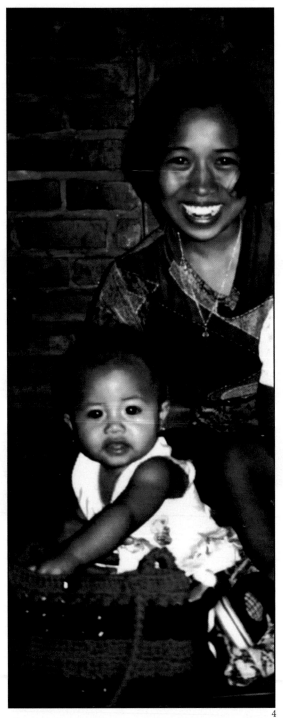

The people of Bali have some of the happiest smiles and kindest hearts of any people I have ever met.

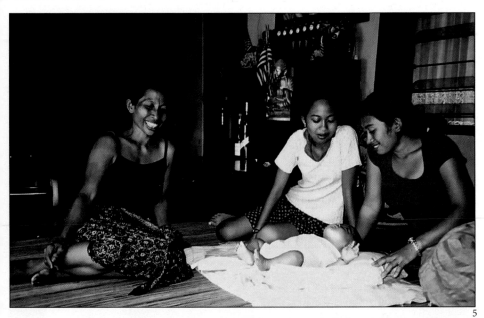

5

Babies in peaceful cultures are never put in another room or left alone; they are always within eyesight of at least one or more loving family members.

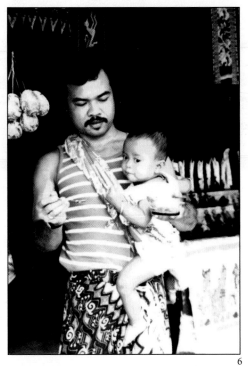

6

Nurturing is highly valued by Balinese men. They are very involved in caring for their children.

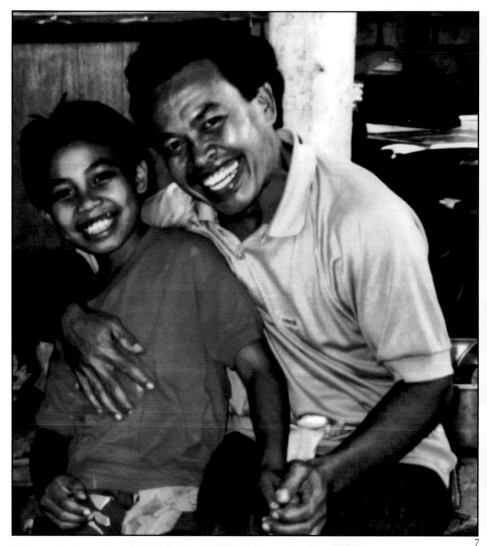

Fathers give lots of attention to their children. It is common to see a preteen son sitting on his dad's lap or a teenager sitting closely with dad's arm around him.

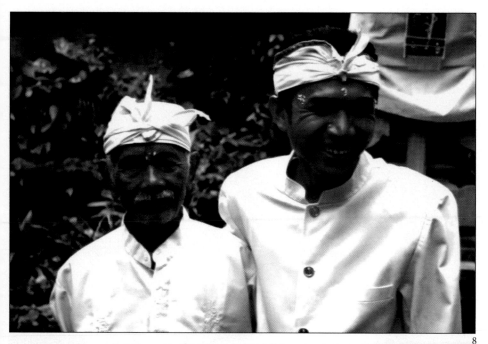

The Balinese know that how we take care of our children in their younger years is directly related to how we will be cared for in our elder years.

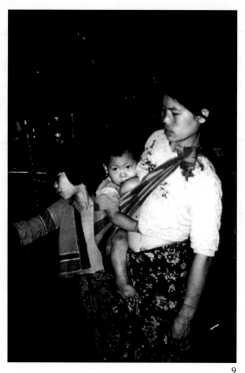

Babies throughout the world are quickly comforted at the breast whenever they desire it.

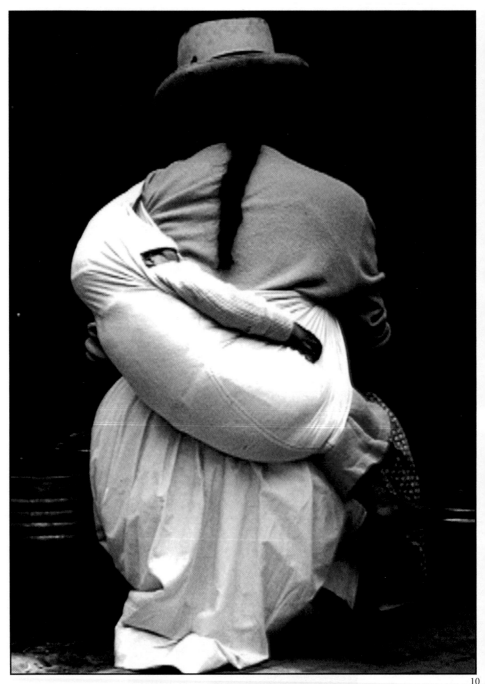

Babies in most of the world are worn on their mom's body and nap there even during their toddler years.

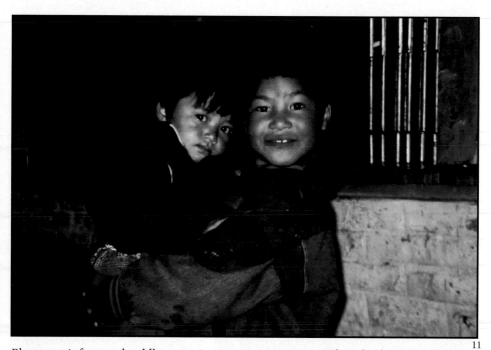

Bhutanese infants and toddlers are given constant attention. When they're not in their parents' arms, they are usually being carried by their older siblings.

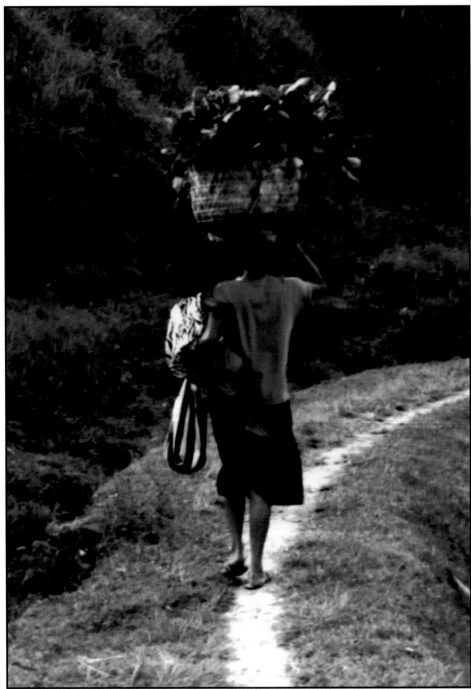

Young children in Bali are usually carried, even if their mom has a heavy load.

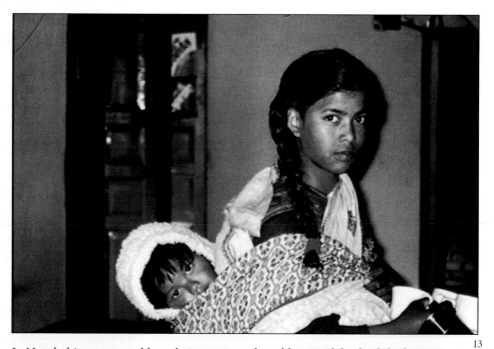

In Nepal, this one-year-old was being worn on her older sister's back while the teen worked as a server in the family restaurant.

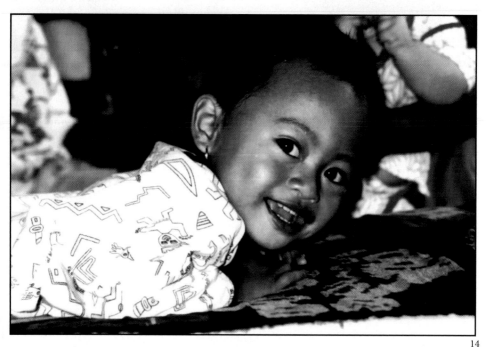

Babies who feel cherished and are given much affection have clear, sparkling eyes that show openness and delight in relationships.

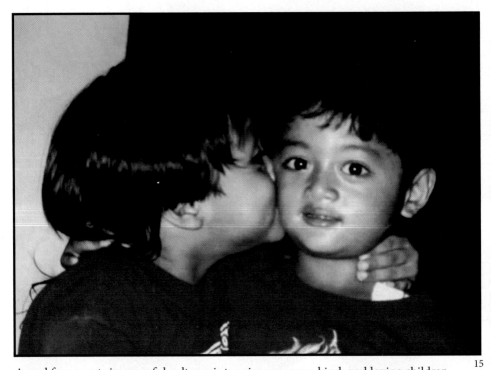

A goal for parents in peaceful cultures is to raise generous, kind, and loving children.

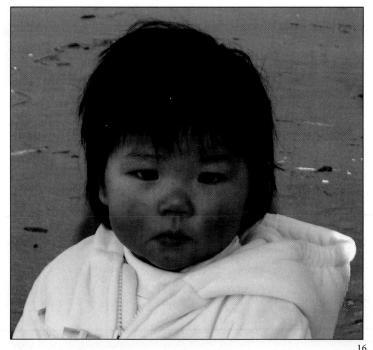

At fourteen months old, four months after being adopted, Julia still[16] had very guarded, shut-down, expressionless eyes.

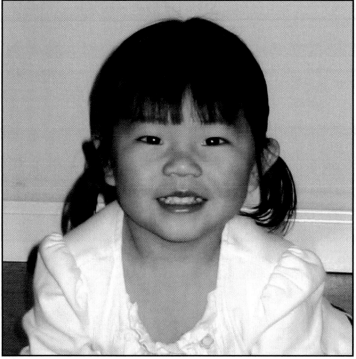

By twenty-eight months, we had been able to entice Julia's little[17] spirit to trust once again.

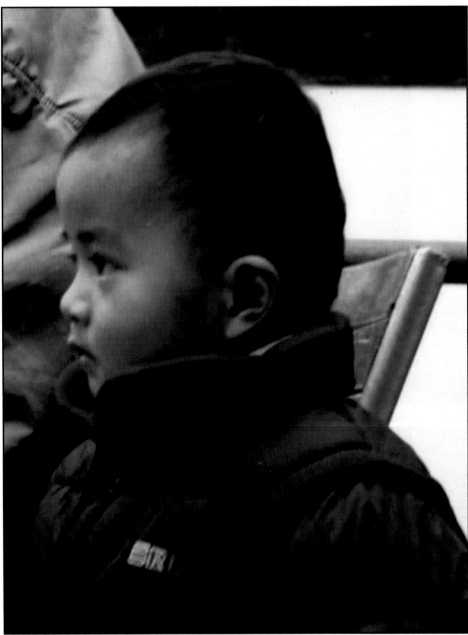

Many toddlers in peaceful cultures have very large protruding foreheads. Could this be due to the growth of larger prefrontal lobes?

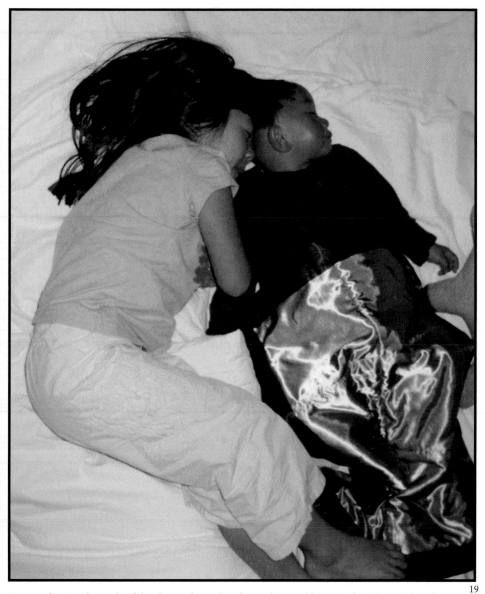

Remembering how she felt when adopted, Julia welcomed her newly-adopted brother warmly, responding lovingly and cuddling him while he slept.

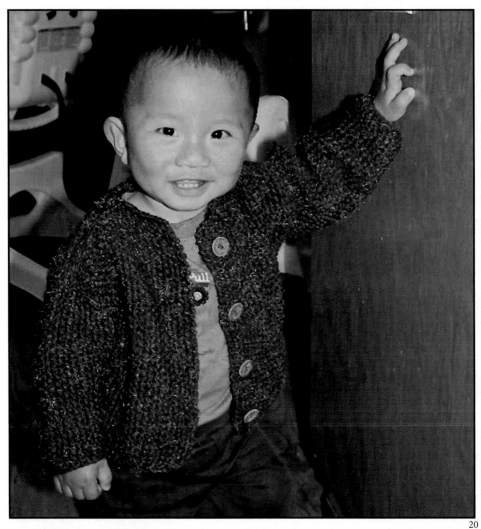

For this little boy, all of the practices that increase attachment were immediately implemented upon adoption, and he was able to "fall in love" with his new family much more easily.

obesity and asthma, along with being six times more likely to have cancer, diabetes, and smoke cigarettes.[27] Bullying is now considered by many to be a significant public health concern.

These early traumatic experiences lead to physical and emotional damage from toxic levels of stress hormones. Poor health apparently comes from discomfort or "dis-ease" within the body; the resulting illnesses depend on inherited sensitivities and the level of stress in children's early environments. The good news is that the opposite is also true: close, secure relationships and a relatively trauma-free early life can contribute to having a healthier mind and body throughout one's lifetime. The early nurturing received by Balinese babies that creates a better ability to naturally produce dopamine in their brains, most likely is the reason these people have historically not used addictive substances. I've been told that there isn't even have a word for addiction in their native language.

---

### Diseases believed to be affected by early life experiences[26]

- Anxiety and Depression
- Addiction to Alcohol, Nicotine and other Drugs
- Alzheimer's disease
- Morbid Obesity and Anorexia Nervosa
- Type 2 Diabetes
- Hypertension
- Irritable Bowel Syndrome
- Ulcerative Colitis and Crohn's disease
- Fibromyalgia
- Osteoarthritis
- Chronic Fatigue and Chronic Pain Syndromes
- Osteoporosis
- Cushing's Syndrome
- Cardiovascular disease
- Susceptibility to Certain Cancers (Including Breast and Melanoma)

## Healing an Attachment-Deprived Child

The degree of nurturing an infant receives shapes the basic structure of the developing brain during the first few years, when it is much more vulnerable to stress. Past belief was that an infant without secure attachment to a significant caregiver in the first year of life would not be able to form trusting relationships throughout his life. However, early brain research has given us far greater hope with the discovery of a process called neural plasticity, which is the ability of the brain to continue adapting to all new experiences over the course of a lifetime.

The window of opportunity for building favorable attachments and healthy social-emotional development is now believed to be at least the first two years after birth. This is especially good news for babies who spend many months without an adequate loving relationship. While healing the brain can continue throughout one's life, if there is too much early deprivation it may never reach its optimal potential.

As a psychologist, I have noticed that children deprived of early nurturing usually have eyes with a distant, guarded, shutdown look that lacks expression. It's as if the connection to their spirits has been diminished or even lost. When I see this look in babies' eyes, I know that work must be done quickly to reconnect them to their feelings and restore their desire and ability to relate to others.

A few years ago, I received a referral from a pediatrician of two worried parents who had adopted a baby from China four months earlier. Although these well-meaning parents were desperately trying to form a loving relationship with their daughter, Julia, she remained detached and distant. The baby had been abandoned at the door of an orphanage when she was just three days old and a week later she was sent to a foster home. At eight months old, she was suddenly taken from that home and returned to the orphanage. Finally, at ten months old she was given to her adoptive parents, who then brought her to the US.

This little baby had experienced the loss of her birth mother, her foster mother, her orphanage caregivers, her home, her country, and even her native language, all before she was a year old. The adoptive parents described Julia as seriously withdrawn, very stressed, irritable with long crying spells, and having great difficulty falling asleep. I noticed that Julia would arch her back and turn away from the parents when they held her. They showed me photos of Julia in China at four months old and on her adoption day at ten months old, and a current photo of her at fourteen months. In all of these pictures, the child had very guarded, shutdown, expressionless eyes (see photo 16). I knew that we didn't have much time to entice her little spirit to trust just one more time.

From my very first session with Julia's adoptive parents, I shared the Global Practices that Increase Attachment (as explained in Chapter 3) and stressed the importance of immediately implementing as many of these as possible.

- Breastfeeding was obviously not an option, but even though Julia was using a cup, I encouraged them to go back to *giving her a bottle* while gently holding and engaging with her. A traumatized baby should never be forced to make eye contact, but should be acknowledged calmly whenever she does eye-gaze using such words as, "Ah, there you are," or "It's so good to see you." Julia's mother reported that the baby was comforted by the bottle feedings and continued wanting them for a very long time.

- Julia's mom got a front pack and even though her daughter was a bit heavy, the mom literally *wore* her child all day long around the house and wherever she went.

- To make up for the lost *skin-to-skin* bonding as a newborn, the parents were encouraged to hold the baby against their skin while lying down, in a rocking chair, in the bathtub together, or wherever she was comfortable with such close contact. A child should never be held in a way that causes anxiety or would discourage feelings of safety and trust.

- *Co-sleeping* was not something that the father was initially willing to try, but her mom began lying close to Julia during naptime. One day when dad saw his wife and daughter sleeping peacefully cuddled up together, it melted his resistance and he knew that something important was happening for Julia, who usually fought going to sleep and had great difficulty staying asleep. (Adopted babies are often transferred while they are sleeping and wake up with strangers in completely unfamiliar places, thereby creating intense fears of falling asleep.) So Julia's parents came up with a compromise. After being rocked to sleep, Julia was placed in her crib; if she awakened, they would go to her. If she seemed scared or couldn't settle back down, they would take her into their bed for the rest of the night. After a short time, they began taking her into their bed *whenever she seemed to need or want to be with them.* They soon noticed how much more comfortable Julia was becoming with them. (In retrospect, these parents believe that bed-sharing was the most important turning point in Julia beginning to attach to them.)

- *Affection* through rocking, cuddling, gentle touch, smiles, and softly spoken baby talk was encouraged as long as Julia was receptive. (She had never even heard the language that was now being spoken to her.)

- The critical importance of *listening and responding* to Julia's cries was vehemently stressed. This baby, who was grieving so many losses, needed to feel understood and comforted by her new parents if she was expected to begin trusting them. Her parents had previously been instructed by their pediatrician and family members not to respond to Julia when she cried during the night. This traumatized little girl had, at times, been screaming for one-and-a-half hours alone in her crib. I had the parents imagine how it would feel to be all alone, terrified, crying loudly for help, and have no one offer comfort. They both instantly understood that this would not help them build trust in any new relationship.

- *Singing* to Julia was one of the most consistently dependable ways of consoling her. Music from China was especially comforting.

- Julia's father was exceptionally good at *playing* with her. And, the more responsive she became, the more he enjoyed their wrestling and tickling games. Whenever Julia awoke from sleep, however, and found one of her parents gone, she would regress into an episode of fearful detachment or inconsolable crying. I suggested they use play as a way to help her understand the new routines of this home and reduce her fear of the unknown. Using a playhouse, small human figures, and a car, they repeatedly showed their daughter which parent was going to work, which parent would be home caring for her, and how the working parent would drive back home at dinnertime. Julia would watch this play and eventually began playing it out for herself; this understanding helped reduce her separation anxiety. I also encouraged the parents never to leave without waking her, telling her good-bye, and reassuring her they would be back.

- The parents made a commitment to continually keep Julia *in close proximity to one of them* and arranged their work schedules so that she could always be with either the mom or dad until she was well attached.

Both parents became very encouraged by their daughter's new willingness to be comforted by them within a few weeks of initiating these parenting practices. Like any relationship, as Julia started opening up to them, they became even more engaged with her. The family began enjoying being with each other and their relationships started growing closer.

While working to help Julia open her heart, each of her parents realized that they had some painful attachment and abandonment issues of their own. Mindful Parenting can definitely trigger our own childhood wounds as we begin to empathize with our children's feelings. In order to be truly openhearted with our children, it is important to recognize how we were hurt as children; otherwise, we tend to unconsciously hurt our own kids in the same ways. Both of Julia's parents were willing to undertake individual and couple counseling to work on their own childhood issues that had left some fears of unconditionally loving each other and their daughter. I was honored to work with these three amazingly resilient people and witness their determination to heal and fully open their hearts to each other. Within fourteen months, it was very clear that Julia's spirit had been retrieved and was clearly showing in her sparkling eyes. As Julia began to heal and trust, her heart opened again and she blossomed into a delightfully caring and lovingly attached toddler (see photo 17).

When Julia was four and a half years old, this family journeyed back to China for the adoption of their son, Leonardo. Parenting skills that helped their little girl heal from her early losses were again called into action, but now the parents had extra help. Julia seemed to remember how scared she had been to lose everyone and everything that had been familiar, and she showed great empathy toward her new little brother. Leonardo did not have to suffer the additional trauma of not feeling understood, as both parents and his sister immediately began engaging in all of the attachment practices that had helped Julia heal. She held her brother gently as she fed him a bottle, tenderly stroked his head, talked soothingly, slept next to him holding his hand, listened to his needs, responded lovingly, sang, played, and delighted in him (see photo 19). The children became closely attached siblings. This is a wonderful example of how the healing of one child can turn into prevention of similar problems for another, just as the healing of one generation prevents passing on those same wounds to future generations (see photo 20). I will always cherish these four people for their hard work and dedication to healing, loving, and creating one of the happiest families I have known, and will be forever grateful to them for allowing me to share their story.

Professionals are still discovering how the power of nurturing affects early brain development and the ways a brain can change, adapt, and heal throughout our lifetime. All humans are born craving unconditional love. Love is our birthright; it is a basic requirement for optimal brain development and leads to a lifetime of health and happiness. If we don't get enough love, it causes emotional damage. Lack of love causes some people to become angrier, some sadder, some withdrawn, some aggressive, some sicker, and some even die. Human hearts and brains are primed to love and be loved even before birth. When babies are welcomed with love, it helps them feel safe and trusting from the beginning of life. Parents are beginning to realize that giving their babies as much love and gentle care as possible from the moment of birth will help them become confident, kind, and loving children.

# CHAPTER 7

# Stresses Faced by Modern Families

*There is more hunger for love and appreciation in this world than for bread.*
*—Mother Teresa*

The balancing of moms' financial and career goals with the needs of their infants and toddlers continues to be an ongoing struggle in this country even forty years after the woman's movement made revolutionary changes in women's lives. While great opportunities were opened to my generation, we were so hungry to be liberated from the housewife-mother roles in which our mothers were trapped that we devalued the importance of caregiving. As we began competing with men for jobs, we tried our best to become more like them. We discounted the need for babies to be nurtured by us, and our need as moms to nurture them.

Unlike our European female counterparts, we tried to do our best at work and at home, both at the same time, and did not even consider asking our employers and governments to help us balance the needs of our babies, families, and careers. European mothers insisted and were granted paid prenatal and postpartum leaves, workplace flexibility, part time jobs with benefits, and quality government-subsidized childcare for their toddlers and older children.[1] Thus they were able to be nurturing moms to their babies and then reenter their careers a few years later with their decently paid jobs waiting for them. American moms, however, wanted to believe that our babies would do just fine being away from us for eight to ten hours a day as long as they were in "quality" day care. As working moms, we were willing to become highly stressed, overworked "supermoms," neglecting our own needs. We tried to prove that we could compete equally with men in the workplace, while still doing our best to care for our children, homes, and husbands. Yes, great progress was made, but we paid the price with symptoms of physical and emotional stress in our babies and ourselves. Our children raised in group-care often became more attached to peers than parents, and our marriages resulted in one of the highest divorce rates in the world.

Current research studies indicate that the stress levels of working moms with young children continues to be many times higher than working dads and may interfere with moms' ability to parent mindfully. Leah C. Hibel of the Department of Human Development and Family Studies at Purdue University has been studying the highly elevated cortisol levels in working moms with children under four years of age. Hibel states with much concern, "The current findings highlight the importance of creating family-friendly policies to reduce the mental, physical, and physiological burden of juggling work and family, especially for mothers with young children."[2]

## Governmental Support for New Families

Nearly every country in the world has built in safeguards that take care of its new mothers through paid leaves during a difficult pregnancy and after the birth of a baby. Of the 188 countries where information about maternity leave policies are known, 181 of them have some form of paid leave for mothers with newborns, with the exception of the United States, Papua New Guinea, Suriname, and a few islands in the South Pacific.[3] (Liberia has recently instituted a paid leave program, so now all countries on the African continent offer such support to new mothers.)[4] Most Americans do not realize that the US is one of the very few countries that doesn't offer *any paid* maternity leave! Even in Saudi Arabia, where women's rights are often minimal, "laws require employers to provide women four weeks of paid leave before their due date, and six weeks of paid maternity leave after delivery."[5] Ninety-eight countries provide at least fourteen weeks of paid maternity leave. Even in developing countries faced with extreme poverty, such as Benin, Cameron, Congo, Ivory Coast, Gabon, Guinea, Mali, Mauritania, Niger, Senegal, Seychelles, and Tonga, those fourteen weeks are paid at one hundred percent of a mother's salary.[6] American mothers are not even given a paid day off to give birth to their babies!

The Nordic countries of Denmark, Finland, Iceland, Norway, and Sweden have a history of being extremely supportive of families. They have goals of maintaining gender equality, supporting career advancement for women, promoting parental involvement for fathers, and ensuring that children have a good start in life.[7]

In Denmark, as soon as women get pregnant they are able to take additional paid sick leave, including extended leave if necessary before the birth and up to a year of paid leave after the baby is born. If there is no father in the home, the government will offer extra "father money" support, and all parents are offered free or highly subsidized quality childcare once a mother returns to work.

In Finland, new parents are given ten months of paid maternity leave, which includes four months specifically for the mother, and the additional six months can be shared between the parents. For the first eight weeks of the leave, mothers receive ninety percent of their salaries. During the remaining eight months, whichever parent is the at-home caregiver receives seventy percent of their salary. *Breastfeeding mothers are allowed up to three years of paid leave* and are then able to return to their same jobs, thus being encouraged to advance in their careers after their babies are weaned. The cost of this paid leave is shared between the employer and the government.[8]

Norway's paid maternity leave is continually being extended and expanded. It now includes paternity leaves in which seventy percent of the fathers are taking part. While in Sweden paid paternal leave has been available since 1995, the current generation of dads is finally taking better advantage of it. Eighty-five percent of Swedish fathers "cannot imagine not using" the two months paid leave that is reserved just for them.[9]

Even though citizens of Nordic countries pay high taxes for such generous family/work policies, they have reaped countless benefits. These programs have contributed to higher productivity, with seventy-five percent of women remaining in the workforce rather than quitting their jobs when they become mothers. Finland prides itself on having the highest student test scores in Europe, and Denmark's citizens are reported to be the happiest in the world.[10] The involvement of fathers in caring for their youngsters has had the accompanying benefit of a lowered divorce rate. Perhaps more marital harmony is created by changing the expectation of mothers being the do-it-all "supermoms," along with dads now understanding and sharing the stresses and joys of caregiving young children. Besides having happier families, parents in Nordic countries don't worry about becoming homeless or being unable to feed their children. Decent wages, paid family leave, flexibility in work schedules, paid sick leave, and government subsidized health care are considered basic rights for all citizens. These countries have the lowest childhood poverty rate in the world, between three and four percent, compared to twenty-two percent in the United States.[11]

Central Europe also has some of the best parental leave policies in the world. France supports new families by giving mothers monetary allocations that encourage women to reduce the number of hours they work during the last few weeks of their pregnancies and one hundred percent of their salaries for the first four months after baby is born. Mothers' jobs are guaranteed back to them for two years and include any pay increases that occurred during her maternity leave.[12] As soon as French toddlers are toilet trained and until they are five years old, ninety percent of them attend free government sponsored nursery schools. These quality childcare programs are staffed by well paid teachers who have had at least two years of college plus two additional years of specialized training in early childhood education. Normally, toddlers attend these preschools for half a day since part-time jobs are regularly made available for the seventy-three percent of young mothers who choose to return to work once their toddlers are old enough to attend the nursery schools.[13] Part-time work for women is also very common in the Netherlands and is gaining popularity among modern fathers. Sixty-five percent of the dads in this generation are much more interested in working less and spending more time with their children. "Part-time work has ceased being the prerogative of [women] with little career ambition, and become a powerful tool to attract and retain talent—male and female—in a competitive Dutch labor market."[14]

Germany has only had a parental leave policy since 2008, when their female chancellor and labor minister fought to make changes. German parents now benefit from fourteen weeks of paid leave at one hundred percent of the at-home parent's salary, an additional fourteen months paid at sixty-five percent, and a remaining year and a half of unpaid leave until the child turns three years old.[15] The mother and father can share this leave as they wish, but the father must take at least two months or those months are lost.[16] This innovative way of encouraging fathers to be more involved as primary caregivers is becoming quite successful.

So, what about other English-speaking countries like England, Australia, and Canada that have conservative and liberal party governments, which are more similar to ours in the US? In 1999, due to the shocking fact that the British had the highest number of children below the poverty line in all of Europe, their government began a twenty-year commitment to end childhood poverty. They instituted a one-year paid family leave policy, six months of which could be used by fathers. Parents received ninety percent of their salary for the first six weeks and twenty-five percent of the national median income for the rest of the year. Kimberly Morgan, associate professor of political science at George Washington University, stated, "I think the idea of family leave soothes the anxieties people might have about mothers' employment and putting small babies in day care because you don't need that if the parent stays home for the first year of a child's life. People feel less nervous about day care when the child is one or two." The British Sure Start program was created to provide all three and four year olds with up to fifteen hours of care per week.[17] Besides bettering the situation for children, British officials believed that providing free quality childcare would improve their economy by making it easier for mothers to return to work, either full or part-time. An innovative "right to request flexibility" program has gotten support from both employers and workers. It allows parents with children under six years of age to request part-time work, flexible scheduling, telecommuting, job sharing, and other ways to adapt to their families' needs. While this flexibility is not mandatory, if the employer refuses to grant an acceptable alternate work schedule, the employee can initiate an appeal process. This creative compromise between the mandated family/work policies of the Nordic countries and the lack of protective policies in the US has proved successful. In England, ninety percent of the requests for flexibility have come from mothers and eighty percent have been granted. Even businesses that vehemently opposed this program initially are now supportive of it, because employers have realized that by being flexible they are able to retain valuable employees.[18]

Australia had a twelve-month unpaid parental leave policy for eighteen years and had a long and difficult fight getting a paid leave policy passed in 2011. All Australians now have eighteen weeks of parental leave paid at the minimum wage of about $16 per hour. A "right to request flexibility" policy similar to that in England has also been adopted.[19]

So, how does our nearby Canadian neighbor support newborns? Maternity leave programs in Canada have been supportive of new families for nearly forty years. All Canadians receive a year of parental leave with their jobs guaranteed back at the end of this time. In most of Canada, the first fifteen weeks are for maternity leave, which is paid at fifty-five percent of the mothers' salaries, up to the limit of $501 per week; the rest of the year is paid at fifty-five percent up to $485 per week, and can be shared between the parents. An even more generous policy exists in the liberal province of Quebec, with twenty-five weeks paid at seventy percent of the parent's salary, up to $835 per week, and another twenty-five weeks at fifty-five percent, up to $656 (thirty-two weeks of this leave can be shared with the father).[20] This one year of parental leave has allowed Canadian parents to be primary caregivers of their infants before returning to their careers. It is important to note that the Canadian economy has not suffered in any way from their support of families, as American business leaders declare would happen if such policies were instituted in the US. Perhaps if infants were given the care they needed, Americans could save much of the tax money that goes to dealing with juvenile problems and housing criminals. The US incarceration rate is the highest in the world, currently nine times higher than in Canada.[21]

Former US Ambassador and Vermont Governor Madeleine Kunin is leading modern American women in the pursuit of greatly needed changes in her recent book *The New Feminist Agenda: Defining the Next Revolution for Women, Work, and Family*. She sums up our current state of affairs in the US by stating that, "not investing in families means that we will continue to fall behind other countries on many yardsticks, from having the highest infant mortality rate among developed countries (forty-seven countries rank better than the US), and the highest incarceration rate, to falling to twelfth place among thirty-six developed countries in the percentage of college graduates . . . Our inability—for political, economic, or cultural reasons—to invest in families leaves us vulnerable to being reduced to second-rate status in the global economy."[22]

## Family/Work Policies in Other Developed Countries[23, 24]

| Country | Length of Paid Leave | Parental Benefits |
|---------|---------------------|-------------------|
| Denmark | 1 year | 100% of salary<br>Paid sick leave during pregnancy<br>2 weeks reserved for the father<br>Extra support if no father in home<br>Free or highly subsidized childcare |
| Finland | 10 months<br>3 years if breastfeeding | 90% of mom's salary for first 8 weeks<br>70% of at-home parent's salary for 8 months<br>4 months for mom and 6 months that parents can share<br>Jobs guaranteed back at end of leave |
| Norway | 3 years | 100% for 10.5 months or 80% for 13 months<br>12 weeks paid leave reserved for father<br>Unpaid maternal leave for additional year<br>Unpaid paternal leave for additional year<br>(Paid paternal leave is used by 70% of dads) |
| Sweden | 16 months | 77.6% of salary for first 13 months<br>Fixed rate for next 3 months<br>2 months are reserved for fathers<br>(Paid paternal leave is used by 85% of dads) |
| France | 2 years | 100% of salary for four months<br>(Increases to 6 months for third child)<br>Free nursery school for 3 to 5 year olds |
| Germany | 3 years | 100% of salary for first 14 weeks<br>(Including 6 weeks before birth)<br>65% of salary for up to 14 months<br>Unpaid up to child's third birthday<br>Can be shared between both parents<br>2 months are reserved for the father |

| | | |
|---|---|---|
| England | 1 year | 90% of salary for 6 weeks<br>25% of median income for rest of year<br>6 months can be used by fathers<br>3 and 4 year olds get 15 hours of care a week<br>Right to request flexibility of employer |
| Australia | 1 year | Minimum wage of $622/week for 16 weeks<br>Unpaid up to 1 year shared between parents<br>Right to request flexibility of employer |
| Japan | 1 year | 60% for 14 weeks<br>Job guaranteed up to baby's first birthday<br>Government funded moms' support groups<br>When parents share, total may be extended up to 1 year for each parent |
| USA | **Unpaid Leave**<br>12 weeks | States where Disability Benefits can be used:<br>California: 55% for 6 weeks<br>Hawaii: 58% (no specified payment duration)<br>New Jersey: 66% for 6 weeks<br>New York: 50% up to 26 weeks<br>New York: 50% |

## Lack of Support for New Families in the US

It has been shown throughout the world that governmental support, which helps parents care for their infants and toddlers, is both good for families and the economy. Family friendly work policies such as paid sick leave, flexibility in work scheduling, and paid parental leave after the birth of a baby, improve the health outcomes for children, reduce employee turnover, and boost both employee performance and loyalty. *The US is the only industrialized country in the entire world that does not have some form of paid governmental leave for new mothers and provides only twelve weeks of unpaid leave.* While there are private businesses in this country that do offer employees some paid leave after the birth of a baby, it is voluntary with the employer covering the total cost, rather than it being shared with the government as it is in most countries.

A new movement is developing in the US in which young workers are requiring family friendly policies from their employers. Forty percent of the current "Millennial Generation Y" parents (those born from about 1982–2000, being the first generation of young adults and children in the new century) say they will leave their jobs if there is not some flexibility in work days and hours, while in the previous Generation X only one third of employees were willing to make such demands; and with the Baby Boomer Generation, it was much less.[25] Fifty percent of "Gen Y" working parents have turned down a job because it would be too hard on their families. Twenty-first century families in the US are very different than in the past: women make up 47 percent of the workforce, 40 percent of moms are either single parents or primary bread earners, and 75 percent of families have both parents working.[26] So, in order for most children to ever have a parent available during the workweek when they become ill, are in a school performance, sports event, or just need some parental comfort, there must be work policies that allow some flexibility. Modern parents want to create a work culture that supports them having more time with their children. They are asserting that their highest priority is to make sure their kids are doing well.

In 2011, the National Science Foundation created a Career-Life Balance Initiative that provides greater work-related flexibility and offers a one-year deferment on previously awarded grants for any employee who needs that time to care for a newborn, newly adopted baby, or to fulfill other family obligations. In June 2014, the American government held its first ever White House Summit on Working Families. Family/work issues were discussed and considerable encouragement was provided for creating changes that will better meet the needs of families. Family friendly policies are repeatedly found to be a win-win for everyone: employees are happier and more productive, thus benefiting employers through increased sales, profit, and growth. It even has been shown that the children of women who are given paid maternity leave grow up to be more productive members of society and earn higher wages later in their own lives.[27]

Besides not having paid sick or parental leaves, many Americans also lack close ties with extended family that include grandparents, aunts, uncles, and cousins to help with hands-on childcare. Instead, we commonly have single mothers or families that are dependent on two incomes, both of which require leaving twelve-week-old infants as long as ten hours each day in large, poorly paid day care facilities. Even middle-income mothers, who can afford to take the allotted period of unpaid leave, find themselves extremely stressed when they are required to return to work and be away from their tiny three-month-old babies all day long. Moms who are worried about their babies can't do their best at work. While the American Pediatric Association recommends exclusive breastfeeding (without any other form of food or liquids) until six months of age, American mothers are only given three months to be home with their babies. This has created a generation of dedicated moms using breast pumps during every one of their work breaks in order for their babies to have the necessary food. As hard as they try, these new moms find it tremendously difficult to keep up with such constant demands. And at the end of the workday, tired, highly-stressed mothers tend to be less patient and respond more harshly to their youngsters. This is unfortunate for moms, because along with all the other things they are worried about, now they have the additional pressure of knowing that their babies, beginning in utero, need their mothers to be less stressed and more nurturing during these first years of life in order to optimize their babies' physical, mental, and emotional development.

It is unnatural for a mother of any mammal to be separated from her newborn. Just as our infants need to feel the connection with their mothers while they are still so very dependent, attached mothers feel an intense instinctive need to be with their babies. There seems to be a lack of understanding in this country that a mother's love and need to care for her infant are natural and should be encouraged. One young mother who was experiencing severe panic attacks when leaving her six-week-old daughter in day care to return to work was recently referred to me for counseling. Her physician had been dismissive of this mom's extreme anxiety, laughingly saying, "Don't worry, honey, you'll get over it." He then prescribed anti-depressant and anti-anxiety medications, which indicated to this new mom that her discomfort with being separated from her infant was a mental disorder! A look of tremendous relief accompanied tears streaming down the young mom's face when I told her that her feelings were completely normal and meant that she had a healthy attachment to her baby. Paid maternity leave should be a basic starting point in any society to encourage and honor the importance of maternal love, attachment, and nurturing for newborn infants.

Some recent polls are showing that a majority of new parents would choose to work part-time and/or have flexible hours if they could make enough money to survive and still maintain such benefits as healthcare.[28] The Affordable Care Act has now made it a reality that no one must stay in a job just to have healthcare. Parents shouldn't need to choose between caregiving their children or having a career; it is time to start advocating for social changes in this country that will help them have both. As US Labor Secretary Tom Perez has beautifully stated to parents, "It's important to put food on the table, but we also want you to be at the table."[29]

## Some States Are Taking The Lead

Until such time that we can count on the US Congress to recognize and support national family-friendly policies, an issue that seems like it should be nonpartisan, appealing to state and local governments for such actions will more likely be successful. A few states, California, Hawaii, New Jersey, New York, and Washington (possibly beginning in October 2015), have become US pioneers in the creation of paid family leave policies using disability insurance to support new mothers and babies. Also, in September 2014, the US Department of Labor awarded $500,000 to provide funding for feasibility studies on paid family and medical leave programs in the District of Columbia, Massachusetts, Montana, and Rhode Island.

California creatively assists new mothers by using their state disability insurance, which is fully funded by employees. The California Pregnancy Disability Leave (CA PDL) provides paid leave beginning four weeks prior to the baby's due date, until six weeks after a vaginal birth, and eight weeks after a cesarean. Mothers receive up to fifty-five percent of their income (to a maximum of $1075 per week in 2014). A woman "disabled" by pregnancy is entitled to four months of disability leave, including time off to recover from severe morning sickness, doctor-ordered bed rest, childbirth, or any other maternal-related medical condition. After a pregnancy disability leave, the woman is guaranteed a return to her same job or if the position is no longer available, a comparable job in terms of pay, location, job content, and promotional opportunities. The California Family Rights Act (CFRA) allows for an additional twelve weeks of unpaid leave to bond with a baby or an older adopted child.[30]

New Jersey adopted a paid family leave law that also uses its employee funded temporary disability insurance program to reimburse for lost wages due to family illness, which can include prenatal and postpartum issues. The law permits an employee six weeks of paid leave to care for a newborn or newly adopted child, or sick parent, spouse, or child. Employees are paid two-thirds of their income (up to a maximum of $524 per week) with their jobs guaranteed back, unless they work for small businesses with less than fifty employees. The most common use of these benefits has been for the care of a new baby, with the next being for the care of an elderly family member.[31]

Hawaiian employers must allow employees to take a reasonable period of leave while they are disabled due to pregnancy, childbirth, and related conditions. The mother's physician determines how long this will be. A mother in New York state is entitled to disability benefits for the period of time that her doctor certifies that she is unable to work, up to twenty-six weeks.

The state of Washington passed a paid family leave law in 2007, but has not yet been financially able to offer these benefits. Washington does not have a disability insurance program and current problems with its economy have not allowed it adequate funding resources, so implementation has been delayed.

About twenty years ago, I approached legislators in my state of Oregon with the idea that, since American parents were not receiving paid parental leaves, maybe low interest state loans could be made available to new parents. Similar to student loans, these parental loans could be obtained by any parent who was staying home full or part-time to care for a child under age six. Perhaps they could also be made available to parents who hire an in-home nanny to care for their baby. The loans could then begin being repaid once the child enters school. It was thought to be "antifeminist" at that time to even suggest that infants and toddlers might need a parent, especially a mother, to care for them. Now that parents are becoming more aware of the importance of being with their babies in those early years, pursuing the possibility of low interest loans should perhaps again be considered. While the recent White House Summit on Working Families was clearly an important first step toward bringing about a federally funded paid parental leave, in the interim, advocating for state or federal low interest loans could be potentially easier and more readily attained.

## Young Couple and Baby Needing Support

The following is a heartfelt story that is a distressing example of why Americans need a higher minimum wage and family-friendly support for new parents including some paid maternity leave to help babies get a healthy start in life. This is an interview with a young mom who unexpectedly discovered she was pregnant, had a difficult birth experience, and received little support from her family. (Planned pregnancies when couples are financially secure and emotionally ready to be parents are certainly the best option, and an optimal beginning for babies as encouraged in peaceful cultures. However, that is not always how it happens, in fact, nearly half of all pregnancies in the US are currently unplanned.) This resilient unmarried couple has forged through many challenging obstacles without ever giving up on love for their daughter or each other. Although their struggles have caused much stress in their relationship and initially challenged the mom's attachment to her baby, they have persevered. But, no matter how hard they have continued to work, it is very hard to get ahead, and this dedicated mom constantly worries about how they are going to meet their daughter's needs and their financial obligations. This baby girl has had to be away from her mom since she was eight weeks old, placed in a poor quality day care; it's a clear example of why the US ought to have much better safety nets to help support babies whose parents can neither afford to take twelve weeks of unpaid leave nor pay for higher quality infant day care. Postpartum depression is all too common in new moms who feel overwhelmed and financially stressed, and is not good for a developing baby's brain. In most other countries this young couple would have had governmental support that would have helped them provide their baby with a more nourishing emotional beginning in life.

*Leslie's Story:*

*When I was twenty-four years old and ready for an adventure in my life, I moved across the country and had been living with my eighteen-year-old partner, James, for only two months when I found out I was pregnant. All of these changes so quickly were quite shocking, and certainly a much different adventure than I'd ever predicted. James and I decided we were going to make it work, but he being in the military, us not being married, living in a small apartment with his mother and stepfather, and me not having health insurance certainly did not make the beginning to my pregnancy an easy one. I was fortunate to get on the Oregon Health Plan after learning that my income combined with James's qualified us for assistance. Thankfully, it paid for my prenatal care, and cesarean birth that was the result of the baby being in a breech position. I had wanted a natural birth, and the doctor-planned C-section with the threat that trying to turn the baby might cause an emergency surgery was mentally hard for me. One regret of mine is that I did not get a second opinion of perhaps a midwife who might have been able to turn the baby successfully, or knew how to deliver it breech. Besides the surgery, I ended up with serious complications including blood clots in my ovaries and severe mastitis. All of this happened at once, plus I never had been a mom, had a newborn to care for, and had no money because I only had unpaid leave.*

*I had no idea what I was doing or what I was going to do. It was so hard and I felt so despondent. I hadn't gone through any labor, which would have at least given me some hormones that could have helped with attachment. I felt like I was cheated out of the birth experience I needed to prepare myself to be a mother, and baby Claire didn't get to pass through the birth canal, which would have given her the stimulation that she needed to be ready for life outside of my body. They just cut her out and put her on my chest; we were both in shock. I felt like my body wasn't ready to have her, yet, and she wasn't ready to be born or to breastfeed, which made nursing always very difficult for us from the very beginning. After Claire was born, I wasn't sleeping at all. I was in too much pain to get around, and couldn't take pain medication without throwing up. I was really struggling and felt like I was drowning. I was thankful Claire was a healthy kid, but for many months I didn't feel really attached to her. There were moments that I felt I wasn't gaining anything positive from this experience of being a mother. I felt like I had screwed up everything and I wondered how I could ever give this baby a good life. It was so hard!*

*Even though James was working all night at a minimum wage job and we were living with his family, it was pretty much impossible to make ends meet. When he got home from work, he really needed to sleep, but I was exhausted from being up with the baby most of the night. The pain from the surgery and complications were still intense. Although James's family did help take care of Claire, it was hard not having any of my own family there. James and I had lots of arguments because it was such a stressful time for us both.*

*Financially I needed to get back to work when Claire was six weeks old, but I still had too much pain and clearly wasn't healed enough. My boss was required by the Family Leave Act to return my full job to me up to twelve weeks after the birth, but even when I tried to return at eight weeks, he told me I could only have thirty hours of work a week because my previous forty-hour job was no longer available. I had to fight to get my unemployment insurance to pay for the additional ten hours per week, which I needed to pay my bills. My boss didn't care about what I was going through and initially even refused to sign the paperwork, saying, "You're the one who decided to take time off." Although I had always considered myself a strong person, I just felt like I was being hit with one thing after another. I felt myself falling into a hopeless depression that I could not pull out of. At least when Claire was about three months old and started making eye contact, cooing, and smiling, I finally began to feel a connection to her.*

*As soon as we got our tax return, we packed up and moved to the Midwest to be near my family. I thought that going back home and being with my mom would fix everything for me. But, when I suddenly showed up in my mom's life with James and the baby, she had a very busy life of her own and couldn't take on the three of us. She did open her home to us for a few months until we sorted out employment and eventually found a place of our own.*

*During the first year and a half of Claire's life she was in a lot of different in-home day care situations. She started going to day care about nine hours a day, three days a week, at eight weeks of age. But for most of her life she has spent at least forty hours a week in day care. There were numerous red flags in many of the day care situations and we pulled her out of lots of them. Working at low paying jobs meant that the day care we could afford was not always adequate. One lady who was caring for Claire and eight other kids in her home didn't seem to be watching her well enough. When we came to pick Claire up she would be in unsafe situations like on the stairs or playing near the toilet. Once she came home with a very bad bruise on her face and the babysitter didn't even know how it had happened.*

*When Claire was eighteen months old, James got a really great job and we were able to get our own place. Things were finally beginning to turn around. At last, I got to be home with Claire, and was able to even take a few college classes. James and I worked out our schedules so one of us could be taking care of Claire, except for just a half-day twice a week of childcare with one of my friends and two other kids. That care at $8.25 per hour was nearly twice as expensive as we'd paid before, but also was much safer and of higher quality. To actually be able to be home with my baby most of the time made this the best period that I've had with Claire since she was born. My depression ultimately lifted. Having time with Claire made so much of a difference; I began to understand her, our communication got so much better, and my relationship with her got so much closer.*

*But after a few months James suddenly lost that job. We sought help once again from my mom, but this time she was adamant that we were old enough to find our own paths. I realized that I couldn't really rely on anyone else, and that James and I would have to make it on our own. We decided, once again, to move back across the country, to at least be where his family was. It really does make a difference that his mom is willing to watch Claire for us if we need a little extra help or wanted a date night together. I appreciate that so much, because being with her grandma is much better for Claire than just having a babysitter. It's very comforting to live near family, and is a security that not a lot of people get to have.*

*Currently, Claire is two-and-a-half years old and with James and I both working full time, Claire goes to day care from 8 a.m. to 5:30 p.m. every weekday for a total of forty-eight hours per week. In the morning it's: get dressed, have breakfast, get in the car, drive to day care, work all day, pick up Claire, come home, make dinner, get ready for bed, and then it's bedtime. On most days I only get to spend three hours a day with my toddler. As a mom it feels pretty heartbreaking. Sometimes I wonder why am I going to work, what is the point of this, it hurts me when I feel that I should be with my child. There's just an instinct there that draws me to be with her. In fact I just told my employer that I want to go down to half-time in the next few months. I don't know how it will work financially, but I know that it's going to help in terms of my sanity. I need more than three hours a day with my daughter to maintain a close relationship.*

*Earlier this year, James didn't have a job and I was working full time. I was fine with that because I felt this was his time to be home with Claire, but he felt like he should be the one working and he didn't want to be at home. Now I'm hoping we can switch that around. I'll be working as a vet tech two days a week and a couple of weekends a month, and do some pet sitting on the side. Now with the Affordable Care Act, I will at least be able to get health insurance, something that I couldn't have done a couple of years ago. I just wish we had some paid family leave so parents could spend more time with their infants and toddlers. And when Claire is in day care, it would be such a blessing to know that trained teachers were actually helping my child develop, rather than her just being "watched" by a babysitter getting less than minimum wage.*

*I feel very fortunate to make $15.25 per hour because so many people make so much less than that. But if I considered having a nanny come to my home, which would be better for Claire, and I tried to pay her a minimum wage, which is $9.10 per hour currently in my state, that would mean I would only be taking home $6.15 per hour to pay for all the rest of the expenses in my life. So many people in this country are getting wages that do not allow them enough money to survive on. It's really tough for my generation. It feels right now like James and I are doing the best we can, but even with both of us working full time, we are still just getting by. We're trying to be good citizens and good parents, but it is really an effort. I feel like I always need to be pro-active and thinking about how to make it all work out, I never feel like I can just relax. Worrying has been the hardest thing about being a mom.*

*My mom worked full time and I pretty much grew up in day care and after school programs. I feel like friends replaced a lot of the attention or connections I was missing with adults. For my whole life I have always been more peer-oriented. My dad was out of the picture after I was six, so it was just my mom. I have a good relationship with my mom, but as a child and adolescent I felt a little detached from her, like I had to take care of myself. When I'd see some of my friends' parents at the school activities, I always felt that my mom was just too busy to do those things. In high school it probably affected me more than it did as a young child, because I was proud of the things I was getting involved in and I wanted her to be there to see them. I definitely want to be more involved in Claire's life.*

*I didn't agree with the way I was raised in which the parent commanded and the child better listen. I always felt a lot of fear when my mom got home because she was stressed out, tired, or angry. I try to remember what it is like to be a kid when an adult is yelling and being crazy and scary. One of the things that I think is most important in terms of being a successful parent is patience and trying to put yourself in the kid's shoes. I'm always trying to blend my mothering with gentleness. I want Claire to be happy when she sees me.*

*Since I've been working full time, I'm glad that I have Wednesdays off to be just with Claire. I always try to do something special with her that is carefree or interesting, something to help us reconnect. This week we went on a nature adventure to some ponds. It's nice getting time to talk with her and have some relaxed fun time together. Sometimes when I'm working on the weekends, I'll take her to work with me and have her help me care for the animals; she loves that.*

*A few weeks ago I took Claire to the library for story time for three to six-year-olds. There was a day care group there and the little kids were trying to get settled and realize they were supposed to listen to the storyteller. When they would get excited about something, the day care workers would give them a sharp snarky command like, "sit and be quiet." The shamed children would gaze downward and it certainly looked harmful to their self-esteems. It made me so sad because I think if their parents knew how their kids were being treated, it would break their hearts. It makes me wonder how many little hurtful things happen each day to Claire that we don't know about.*

*Even though James and I had some difficult times, we still enjoy being together and have managed to create balance in our lives. Our favorite time to just be with each other is after Claire goes to bed. We don't let being parents stop us from having fun, and go on many adventures together as a family. Initially I tried to control everything, but I realized that James was trying to figure out how to be a father and I needed to let him do that. I'm still learning and there are times that I want to correct him about how he is dealing with Claire, but I know I need to step down at those times. He doesn't need to be parented by me, and overall he's done a really good job taking care of Claire and me. James is definitely a hands-on dad and even cooks most all of the meals. Both of us have foundered at times and there certainly were bursts of frustration and anger, but we remember how much we have gone through together and it has made us feel stronger as a couple. I know I can depend on James to help me in the worst situation of my life, and I have also shown him that I will always stand up for him. James is very giving, warm-hearted, and does a good job of keeping the love alive. I don't know what I would do without him.*

## Relationship Stress Between Parents

The birth or adoption of a baby and the few years following the addition of that child into the family is one of the most stressful times in couples' relationships. While parents may experience increased personal happiness, comfort in their relationship is frequently at an all-time low. Finding ways to alleviate relationship strains will help create a happier family and a more positive environment for the baby's developing brain and feelings of security. Tension between parents often stems from exhaustion, anxiety, isolation, financial stresses, greatly diminished sex drive in lactating women (evolved to prevent another conception until infants and toddlers are much less dependent), lack of time to have fun together, and rivalry between the two parents concerning care of the baby.

Typically, moms, due to their intense interconnection from pregnancy, birth, and breastfeeding, experience such strong synchronicity with their infant that they feel the way they are caring for their baby is the right way, and they often correct the dads repeatedly telling them they are doing

things wrong. This obviously does not encourage involvement, cooperation, or harmony in their relationship. Of course, if something is harmful,
moms need to speak up, but usually it is just that dads do it differently.
One big difference is that moms tend to be more quiet nurturers while
dads tend to love the more rough and tumble play. Babies truly benefit
from having both parenting styles as each provides a uniquely important
dynamic to their lives. In the peaceful cultures, dads and moms tend to
appreciate and value what they each offer their child. As in any team, it
helps to have players with differing skill sets. Viewing yourselves as being
on the same team can go a long way to create positive feelings in your
relationship and provide your baby with a richer array of life experiences.

Another area of contention in many couples is around breastfeeding.
Moms obviously have an instant way to comfort a screaming baby at the
breast that can make even the most supportive dads envious at times.
There is a mistaken belief that a father needs to feed his baby bottles of
breast milk in order to develop a closer bond. Actually, a dad that encourages the breastfeeding relationship and quickly hands the unhappy baby
to her mother will most likely in the long run have a closer relationship
with both of them. The baby feels most comforted at the breast and the
mom is spared from unnecessary breast pumping, a less than optimal
experience. This is not to say that it isn't sometimes helpful or necessary
for a father to feed the baby from a bottle, but it isn't necessary to promote
a closer attachment. While moms can easily pacify a crying baby by nursing, dads can find their own creative ways to comfort or playfully change
a baby's mood. For example, skin-to-skin, baby wearing, and playtime
with a dad will go a long way in keeping their connection a close one.

Many moms are resentful that their partner's body and life has not
changed as much as theirs have. And some dads feel abandoned in those
early years when moms are so involved with caring for their babies. Those
dads who didn't get much nurturing as babies themselves can feel jealous of the attention their partner is giving to the baby. "Witnessing his
child suckling at the breast, being lovingly held in arms, and receiving the
attention and nurturance he craves, can be devastating to a new father."[32]
Those moms and dads who understand that these feelings are normal,
can communicate that they are both feeling jealous of the other at times,

and disclose that they often miss and want more attention from each other, can create a shared experience that brings closeness rather than distance. Parents who express their appreciations of each other (something we all desperately crave) and make sure there is always time to be playful and laugh together help increase resiliency in their relationship. It can be healing and inviting to realize that by working together, they are creating a family bond that can be even stronger and more rewarding than that which they shared as a couple.

Understanding that they are giving their baby something extremely valuable that they wish they had gotten as children can turn feelings of resentment into ones of open heartedness. A new opportunity and second chance at having the parent-child bond and happy family they may have always wished for now exists with them as the parents in charge. Hands-on dads who realize what an important role they play in their partner's and baby's lives have enhanced feelings of love, loyalty, and commitment to their families that will hopefully create a generation with happier couples and many fewer broken homes.

## Day Care vs. Home Care

One of the most controversial issues for new parents is whether day care, which has become commonly used in the US, is harmful for infants and toddlers. While day care may be helpful to parents who are struggling to make it financially and for those dedicated to their career, it has never been shown to be good for babies. Family psychologist Steve Biddulph has aptly stated, "Childcare was not invented for children's sakes, but for adult needs."[33] How potentially harmful it is to babies continues to be debated, but most of the numerous international studies conducted, to the dismay of many, have shown that babies cared for out of their homes by nonrelated providers experience high levels of stress that can be damaging to emotional, social, and psychological development. Many of these studies have had a hard time getting published and the findings are often distorted because no one wants to make well-meaning already stressed parents feel guilty about their childcare choices. Parents, however, deserve to have all information that is available when it comes to issues that affect decisions they are making for their children. My observation is that parents' awareness of what their babies truly need is creating a new movement in which millions of parents are jumping on board to help change the current system in which American parents are neither supported nor given time to be with their infants and toddlers.

There are two major types of research regarding the impact of day care on babies. Some studies look at the long-term emotional and behavioral impact of childcare over many years, and more recent studies are testing the stress hormone cortisol in babies, which can be damaging to their young developing brains. (See Chapter 6's Parenting for Optimal Brain Development)

The National Institute of Child Health and Development (NICHD) has been conducting a long-term study that started in 1990 and is still in progress. It began in ten US cities with 1,364 infants at one month of age from rich and poor, single and two-parent families. Some findings, to date, are that longer hours in day care affect the sensitivity and harmony of the mother-infant relationship, and that the greater the number of hours spent in day care, regardless of quality, the higher the rate of aggression and behavioral problems in those children by the time they reach kindergarten.[34]

It was shocking to me when I calculated that infants who are commonly left in day care each weekday from 7:30 a.m. to 5:30 p.m. for fifty weeks per year spend twenty-five hundred hours in care, which is more than twice as many hours as six-year-olds spend in first grade during a school year of 1,080 hours (9:00 a.m. to 3:00 p.m. for thirty-six weeks).

Two studies in Great Britain, one in Northern Ireland, and one in California have all shown similar findings in terms of difficulties with socialization and increased anxiety among children who spent long hours in day care when they were under two years of age.[35] Anne Manne, Australian author of the book *Motherhood*, concludes that after thirty years of controversy, at least three major reviews of research have confirmed a direct correlation between extensive time spent in day care centers and higher rates of insecure attachment in infants. Trouble with attachment leads to long-term difficulties in solving problems, regulating emotions, trusting others, and having successful future relationships. Manne also reports the results of a study that researchers had a very difficult time getting published, which found that infants who had spent thirty or more hours per week in day care scored lower in work habits, emotional well-being, peer relationships, and overall compliance when they were third graders.[36] In Canada, a meta-analysis of all studies conducted in Western countries since 1957 revealed that "when young children spend more than twenty hours a week in day care, there is a negative effect on attachment, behavioral adjustment, and social-emotional development compared to children who are cared for at home."[37]

The American experiment with having children attend full-time day care from the first few months of life until they enter school full time at age six is now nearly forty years old. If this experiment had been successful, it doesn't seem reasonable that we would have the childhood emotional distress, which we are experiencing in this country—with twenty percent of kids being diagnosed with a psychological disorder; using ninety percent of all medications in the world that are given to children for mental health issues; having a high and growing child suicide rate; and a greatly increased incidence of bullying, in which children are even killing other children.

Unfortunately, group care outside the home, which has become widely accepted and thought to be a necessity for many working parents, does not appear to be a healthy option for many infants and young toddlers. Some people question whether it is detrimental for infants not to be in day care where they can learn to socialize with other children. Parents need not worry about that because children do not learn to play with other children until they are about three years old. This is the reason that preschools in most developed countries start at that age. Three-month-olds need much different care than three-year-olds. In addition to babies needing a one-to-one nurturing relationship during the first few years of life, babies can also experience overstimulation in day care due to the high energy and needs of the other children. British psychologist Penelope Leach, who has written extensively on parenting issues from the perspective of child development reports, "It is clearly and certainly best for babies to have something close to full-time mother care for six months at least, conveniently linked with breastfeeding, and family care for a further year and better two."[38]

In the peaceful cultures with the current generation's commitment to only have a couple of children, there are normally a ratio of four adults in large extended families helping care for each infant. Even in the best of American day cares, the ratio is usually the opposite, approximately four babies cared for by each adult. If we consider how overwhelming it would be to take care of four infants at the same time, we owe great gratitude to those dedicated caregivers who try their best. Ask any mother of twins if she could easily add another set of twins to her already exhausting day and successfully meet the babies' needs. I know how difficult it was for my own mother who had twins when I was fourteen months old to care for three babies all at once and am exceedingly thankful that my grandmother was there to help.

Until the US has some paid parental leave, it is important to consider what qualities a state-of-the-art dedicated baby day care program would look like. The staff at the Vivian Olum Child Development Center on the University of Oregon campus has put great effort into trying to reduce the stressful impact of day care on babies. Twenty years ago, Dr. Vivian Olum, a beloved professor of child psychology at the university, was concerned about infants being in day care. Since infant day care was becoming a common practice, a center was dedicated in Dr. Olum's name with the promise of trying to comprehend, identify, and provide developmentally for the emotional and physical needs of babies.

The Vivian Olum Center's infant program is limited to eight babies from eight weeks to a year old whose parents make a one-year commitment at their annual September enrollment, thereby creating a stable group in which each baby's needs and temperament becomes well known. Their two highly qualified teachers make long-term commitments to the program, and they try to stay with the same group of babies for at least two to three years as they move into the toddler program. University students work in the program for ten to fifteen hours a week, which nicely reduces the teacher-baby ratio, and they are often willing to do some in-home babysitting after-hours for the infants they've come to know. Before an infant enters the day care program, one of the teachers makes a home visit to become acquainted with the parents' and baby's routines in their own environment. Then begins a slow transition from home care to day care with only half the infants starting the first week and being there only for half-days. The second week, the next four babies begin attending only half-days, while the group from week one now stays full-days. Parents "practice" leaving and coming back many times during those first few weeks and are then encouraged to visit as often as they can. Most of the babies are still breastfeeding with mothers who usually come to feed them a few times a day. The staff is well trained in all areas of infant development. They continually alter the room arrangement and toys to meet the quickly changing needs and interests of the rapidly developing babies throughout the year to keep it a stimulating environment. When a particular baby is having difficulty, for instance with separation, the parents and staff meet to brainstorm ideas such as leaving a piece of mom's clothing that comfortingly smells like her. Since parents always feel welcomed, they begin forming relationships with each other during their visits. It is common to see them gathering outside on the grassy campus area to talk with each other and play with the babies after hours.

While all attempts are made at the Vivian Olum Center to mindfully meet the needs of the babies, staff members readily point out that this is nevertheless "center-based care," rather than home care, which is still more optimal for infants. In spite of everything that is done, the environment is often difficult for babies, who are separated from their parents and don't have moms' comfort nursing when it's needed. Particularly distressed are those who are especially sensitive to sound and energy, becoming overstimulated by so many other babies and adults in the room. It is reported that there are lots of crying babies, especially during the first few weeks. While university student caregivers agree to stay throughout the year, their lives often change making that not an option, which is additionally hard for babies who have become attached to them. This type of attentive infant care is also very expensive, even though the teachers are still underpaid relative to the demands and importance of their jobs, and despite the fact that parents pay a premium, the university still has to subsidize this program.[39] Most other governments have concluded that instead of spending resources trying to develop high enough quality infant day care, the investment in helping infants receive care from their own parents through paid parental leaves is more cost beneficial, better for babies, and in the long-term better for their societies.

Many people have questioned whether I should mention that day care is not best for infants and toddlers, because it may make parents feel guilty about something they can do nothing about. It is certainly true that many parents, especially those in low-paying jobs, need to have their baby in day care; they don't really know of any other options. Even if they are a two-parent family, it can be very hard to make ends meet. The average minimum wage has decreased in value twenty percent in the past thirty years.[40] Although parents want what is best for their babies, they also have a lot of other worries and concerns. Inducing guilt is absolutely not something I want to inflict on parents who are working so hard to meet their children's needs. I believe that guilt comes from intentionally doing something you know might be hurtful, while regret comes from wishing one had known differently or had other options available. As a nation, we should feel guilty that we are not helping parents the way they deserve to be supported, and my heart truly goes out to all those parents who desperately wish that other options were available. While I know it will be difficult to hear that day care may be potentially harmful to infants and toddlers, my wish is that it can also offer support to those parents who are already feeling uncomfortable about this issue, and perhaps offer them a ray of hope that others are listening and that change is coming.

Understandably, there will always be a need for some type of childcare for babies who have single parents, families that need two incomes to meet their basic expenses, and those without the desire or ability to care for an infant all day long (not all people are good at that job). The next chapter offers these parents options besides group day care that may more favorably meet their infant's needs along with taking into consideration parents' own needs as individuals, couples, and families.

# CHAPTER 8

# Modern Parents:
# Balancing Careers and Children

*Just remember that a hundred years from now,*
*It won't matter what your bank account was,*
*What sort of house you lived in, or the kind of car you drove,*
*But, the world may be different,*
*Because you were deeply involved in the lives of your children.*

*—Anonymous*

Evidence from peaceful cultures and early brain research reveals that infants and toddlers who receive consistent attention and affection by attached, nurturing caregivers during their first three years of life emotionally blossom into happy, resilient, and loveable children. My first pregnancy occurred soon after returning in the mid-seventies from fourteen months of observing the contentment of babies in indigenous South American cultures. Knowing I wanted to incorporate their gentle nurturing practices, I modeled most of my early mothering after what I had witnessed. I also decided to spend the first year with my baby as an at-home mom.

I regret, however, that when Shane was fourteen months old, my career goals, lack of extended family support, and the acceptable American child-rearing practices of the day led me to choose a well-respected day care option for my little son. My content, confident, smiley little baby was not ready to be suddenly left with a handful of strangers caring for a roomful of babies, even though the ratio of adults to babies was considered "optimal" at one to four. I watched sadly as Shane became fretful and clingy, began having difficulty sleeping, and became fearful when I even walked into another room. After a few weeks of hoping that Shane would "adapt," we eventually moved him to an in-home day care with a grandmotherly woman who was also caring for a couple of other children up to age five. In addition, Shane's dad changed his work schedule in order to spend some afternoons at home with him. While Shane did do better with that arrangement, his delightfully joyful, totally trusting personality never seemed to fully recover. I wish I had realized that he needed another couple of years of consistent nurturing by his mom, dad, or a loving caregiver in our own home.

Although I understood the importance of attachment and trust in relationships that resulted from receiving one-to-one nurturing care as an infant, the brain research supporting the continuation of such care during the toddler years was not yet available. Nor did I fully reflect on the fact that I had decades in the future to be career oriented, but only a few years to build a strong emotional foundation for my child. After all, I had spent ten years studying to become a psychologist; couldn't I have given my son at least three years of security before heading back into my career? At that time, American women were fighting hard for educational and career opportunities, and the idea of professional women being "at-home moms" was a totally foreign concept. It felt like I had to choose between either being a stay-at-home mom or pursuing my professional goals; I didn't consider that I could do both. In fact, even during my year at home I was often confronted with raised eyebrows, snide comments, and the dreaded disapproving question, "Are you *just* staying home with the baby?" Hopefully, a new understanding is developing that spending the first few years caring for your babies is the most important and challenging job that parents can do in terms of raising emotionally healthy, self-confident, and compassionate children.

When my daughter Emily was born, eight years later, I was determined not to make the same mistake again, even though there was much pressure from my husband, colleagues, and friends to get back to work as soon as possible and give infant day care another try. I held out once again for nearly an entire year at home with Emily, but then grudgingly returned to work a few days a week. By that time, Emily's dad was busy in the productive years of his profession, being the primary financial provider for our family, and was no longer willing to spend afternoons at home. I was determined that Emily would be cared for in our home by a primary caregiver to whom she could form a close relationship.

I found a delightfully loving college student nanny, who cared for our neighbor's children, to do in-home one-to-one care of Emily until she was three years old. At that point Emily was ready for a half-day of preschool socialization and the nanny cared for her after preschool on my three workdays per week. Our nanny and her equally baby-loving sister continued to care for Emily whenever we needed help throughout the rest of Emily's childhood and are still very important people in her life. After the toddler years, the neighbor and I would sometimes arrange to have one of the nannies care for all our kids together. The two nanny sisters often met with both of us moms to consult about how the kids were doing. Family-type relationships developed as we began sharing birthdays, holidays, and other special events. When our daughters got older, they wanted to join in our mom-nanny meetings. And when the nannies later became mothers themselves, their babies were often cared for by our daughters. After thirty years, our three generations of women, now including our sons' partners, are known fondly as the "Soul Sisters," who meet often and share a close, loving bond. Although I still regret not delaying my return to work until Emily was older, she clearly fared well with these extended family-type arrangements.

Today's "Millennial Generation Y" parents are earnestly searching for answers as to how they can best meet the emotional needs of their youngsters. This generation is the first to have grown up spending the majority of each day away from both their parents because of dual careers and single-parent families. Many of these young adults remember feelings of anxiety and loneliness from their childhoods. Most of them believe that peers became their closest relationships and that they missed out on something important in terms of closeness with their parents, grandparents, and extended families. These memories are spurring a new social movement in parenting. Modern parents are challenging the old assumption that the quality of time spent with children is more valuable than the quantity of time. They understand that the times when our kids need us most don't fit into rigid schedules, and being available to our babies during the first few years is what matters most to their sense of security and trust in relationships. Fathers of this generation definitely want to be more involved in their children's lives. The Pew Research center reports that dads today spend more that twice as much time doing household chores and triple the time caring for their children than men did fifty years ago.[1] As parents are becoming aware of infants' and toddlers' emotional needs and how babies in other countries are getting those needs met, they are beginning to demand changes. In the previous generation, we spoke up for women's rights; this generation is beginning to speak up for children's rights.

In an attempt to meet the changing needs of young children, it helps to view parenting as having different stages. Infants are least stressed when their first nine months (the second half of their gestation) can be with the mother in whom they gestated; they then are able to feel secure with their involved fathers, grandparents, nannies, or other attached caregivers. A three-year-old can benefit from preschool socialization with other toddlers, and a six-year-old is ready to be away from her parents for an entire school day. Honoring children's needs at these different stages is what youngsters are commonly receiving in other countries.

"Millennial" parents are beginning to ask employers and elected officials for policy changes that can help working families better provide for their kids' needs. While parents living from paycheck to paycheck in minimum wage jobs may not be able to risk asking their employers for more family supportive policies, parents in career positions that provide more job security can advocate for all parents by requesting such changes. Although family friendly workplace attitudes are slowly developing, modern parents are also creating their own unique ways to meet their babies' needs.

Included in this chapter are personal interviews from parents of Gen Y who are making outstanding changes in the ways their babies are being cared for, while at the same time striving to meet their financial, career, and household responsibilities. My hope is that these stories, which I found tremendously inspiring, will offer parents new possibilities never before considered or perhaps help stimulate their own creative options. All of the parents interviewed clearly understood the importance of maintaining a close relationship with their babies and whenever they felt disconnected, they worked extra hard to reconnect with them. These parents were willing to share intimate details of their greatest joys and most difficult personal and relationships challenges that came with having a baby in their lives. It was heartwarming to hear how many of them had created supportive communities with other new parents in order to help each other in this all-encompassing job of childrearing. These stories are written just as they were told to me, except everyone's name was changed to protect their privacy.

Never underestimate the power of parents when they know their babies need something changed in order to be healthier. Just think of how mothers radically went back to breastfeeding once they realized how important it was to their baby's health and well-being. Similarly, parents who are now becoming aware of the importance of prolonged infant nurturing are beginning to require that employers and legislators provide family/work policies that will help them meet those needs. The US Secretary of Labor, Thomas E. Perez, has recently stated that no parent should "have to chose between the job that they need and the family that they love."

## Creative Ways to Meet Babies' Needs

Providing mindful, responsive care to a mother and baby during the postpartum period results in stronger attachment, increased nurturing, longer-term exclusive breastfeeding, a lower rate of infant mortality, and improved brain development. It is clear that babies want to continue the relationship that began in the womb, and most closely-attached new mothers want to be with their infants. Something that is making it a bit easier for moms of this generation is that they generally aren't as driven to attain the "supermom" status of the past, when moms tried to do it all, and all at the same time. In fact, there is a newly emerging movement encouraging women to divide their lives into three distinct developmental stages. The decade of their twenties can be focused on education (meeting career goals), exploration (such as travel, self-awareness, and adventure), and dating (to discover a good match for their life-partner). The main focus of their thirties is then on marriage, pregnancies, early child rearing, and creating a healthy foundation for their families, while keeping aware of changes in their careers through working part-time, attending conferences, and networking. Since we are living longer healthier lives, this leaves their forties, fifties, sixties, and even seventies to devote more time to their long-held career advancement goals. While life can throw unexpected challenges into even our most well thought-out plans, having such a basic outline of priorities can reduce anxiety, help women be more proactive, and provide extra resilience when they get thrown off track.

However, even if we had one to three years of paid maternity leave in this country, not all women have the desire or patience to be at-home-moms. My own mom seemed stressed and unhappy caring for five children, so even though she was at home, it wasn't really a positive experience for any of us. Sometimes the most loving caregiver could be the dad, grandmother, grandfather, another family member, a friend, or a nanny. One good test of whether someone would be a good caregiver for your baby is to ask yourself: if you were suddenly completely dependent, unable to talk, walk, or even scratch an itch, and needed someone to care for your body, heart, and mind, who would you feel safe and comfortable being left with for ten hours a day, five days a week? Of most importance for your infant is that the chosen primary caregiver is attentive, gentle, and delights in caring for your baby.

Millennial parents have developed some amazingly creative alternatives to using day care especially during their children's first three most formative infant and toddler years. These parents are making reassuring changes to help babies get more hands-on nurturing while also creating happier families. Their determination and flexibility in adapting their lifestyles to meet the early needs of their babies is inspiring. These changes include: simplifying their lives in order to reduce the financial burden, choosing one of the parents to be at-home for the infant and toddler years, involving more extended family support, and/or using grandparents, friends, or nannies as primary caregivers. Most parents I interviewed were using an innovative combination of nearly all these options. Gen Y is clearly forging new paths, breaking down barriers, and persuading employers and their own family members to be supportive in helping them raise healthy, capable and kind kids.

## Simplify Your Lives

*The best things in life aren't things.*

—Art Buchwald

A cultural norm in the US has been based on working hard to get money to buy things. Unfortunately, there is often a strong desire to have things that we can't afford, resulting in the need to work even harder to get more money to pay off those bills. We then continue buying more things that we can't afford, creating the need to work even harder, and so it continues. While this may be good for credit card companies and big businesses that are raking in money, it causes much stress to wage earners and their families. Even middle-class parents who have two good incomes can become accustomed to having a lifestyle in which they continually purchase more things. What was once nonessential slowly becomes essential and the consumption bar continues to be raised, causing wage earners to constantly strive harder to achieve the same level of satisfaction. In our struggling economy, today's parents are faced with the old battle between time and money even more than their parents were. This cycle of wanting and needing causes increased stress in great numbers of Americans, often leading to troubling levels of anxiety. Anxiety has become the most common mental disorder in the US, affecting forty million adults and often accompanied by depression and other stress-related illnesses.[2]

It has been difficult in the past for Americans to simplify their lives once they became parents. The tendency has been to keep working just as hard in their jobs while multitasking the responsibilities of their home and the caregiving of their children. Constant striving, even when it causes them more stress, does not make anyone in the family happier. This is different from the lifestyles of Europeans who are opting for more time than money, desiring four-day workweeks and longer vacations to spend with their families, or the people in the peaceful culture of Bhutan in which the concept of Gross National Happiness is more important than Gross National Product.

The definition of "simplify" means to "make something easier." One of the ways that some modern parents are trying to meet the needs of their infants and toddlers, along with making their lives easier, is to cut back on their expenses. Infants do not really care if they have bigger houses, expensive cars to ride in, fancy baby furniture, state-of-the-art toys, or designer clothes; all they really want is to have a loving parent meeting their needs and playing and delighting in being with them. While having enough money to meet our basic needs is important, the second thing that most promotes human happiness is time spent enjoying activities with family and friends. Mindful parents seem to be realizing that enjoying more time with their children at the beginning of their lives will make for a happier family and ultimately save money, because building a healthy emotional foundation in your children will allow them to become more self-sufficient and resilient in dealing with later life challenges.

Parents are often pleasantly surprised at how much less money they need when having an at-home parent. The biggest savings is usually from not paying day care expenses (average cost of about $1000/month), but money is also saved by not needing to buy new work clothes, lunches and dinners out, gas money driving to/from day care and work, perhaps not needing two cars, etc. These expenses add up to a significant amount of money that the parent working outside the home does not need to earn. Most of the families that opt for a stay-at-home parent are able to do this by greatly simplifying their lifestyles so they can live on one income.

## Same Gender Couple Simplified Their Lives

*Callie's Story:*

*When my wife, Lesley, and I decided to have kids, we agreed that due to our bodies and personalities, I would be the one to carry our babies. Lesley was afraid that as an older mom, if she were pregnant she might not feel well enough for the focused responsibilities in her new profession. I was fortunate that even being thirty-seven and thirty-nine years old when the kids were born, I had very easy pregnancies. Since Lesley had the better paying job and I would be breastfeeding, it made sense that I'd be the at-home mom. Lesley and I had seriously talked about our financial pri-*

orities and set up our household so that we could live on her income from the time our kids were born through preschool. We made conscious choices never to build up debt, to have used cars and hand-me-down clothes for the kids that we would happily to pass on to others, and, most importantly, to live in a modest house, making sure our mortgage was very doable. The bottom-line most important decision we made was not to live in a house that was beyond our means. Even later when we did a bit of remodeling, we always made sure we could comfortably afford our mortgage. This is the biggest reason we have been able to live the life we've had without me working while the kids were young. Lesley and I realized early on that we couldn't afford the kinds of vacations we used to take, so when our first baby, Ellie, was itty bitty, we got a port-a-crib and decided to do lots of camping. We had a group of friends who would camp in the same campground with us every summer at the coast. We have great memories of all the little kids spending time playing in the creek and on the beach. Many of our friends with two professional incomes take trips to Hawaii every year, but we've accepted that if we ever wanted a vacation like that we'd need to save up for at least four years. Even as the kids have grown, we've kept to our original plan to simplify our lives in order to have more time as a family.

I breastfed both babies for a year, but would always pump enough milk so that when Lesley got home from work, she could do the bedtime feeding. Pumping is a lot of work, but it seemed especially important to Lesley to have that connection of feeding the babies. I think any parent who has to be away from their babies really misses them. I can't even imagine how hard it would have been if I had not been able to be with the babies all day long. But Lesley trusted that I was doing a good job with the kids and that gave her a sense of comfort. It was sorta a classic type arrangement in which Lesley was the financial provider, and besides taking care of the kids, I always had dinner ready when she got home. Every night we sat down and ate together with the babies right at the table with us. When Lesley was at home, she was good at leaving work behind and being an involved mom. Because she was working so hard, I would get up during the night when the babies needed care during the week, but on the weekends Lesley would take the night shift, bringing the babies to me to be nursed.

*When the kids got older, Lesley usually had one of her days off during the week and she would spend that time with the kids, even volunteering at their schools. It seemed especially important to us as a lesbian couple to have Ellie and Joey's classmates see us as a family. In fact, I think it would be really great if all parents could have more flexible hours so they would have a day off during the week to be more involved in that part of their kids' lives.*

*Lesley and I went into the decision to have children very thoughtfully, it took great planning; a pregnancy certainly couldn't happen for us by accident. We thought a lot about how we wanted those early years to be. The fact that we were a lesbian couple didn't really make much difference when the kids were babies. We were just two parents in our own home doing what every other family with babies was doing. But we knew that nothing would "out" us more than having kids. We could not be ashamed of who we were in the world or hide our lifestyle because that discomfort would only damage our children. So, in a way, the kids have been the gift that helped Lesley and I say, "This is who we are, and we are a family." We joined a Birth To Three group and other groups with both gay and straight parents rather than the Rainbow Rascals parenting group of just gay and lesbian families. We have always felt accepted and didn't want to start our kids off in a segregated group. We wanted the kids to always feel included in the much larger world.*

*When Ellie was nearly three years old and started preschool, all of a sudden I felt very vulnerable. I was worried about how other parents' opinions and feelings about us being lesbians would affect Ellie since this was the beginning of her experience out in the world. We were careful about choosing a city and neighborhood where we thought we'd be welcomed. But when it's your kids, you worry about whether they'll be accepted. The school was actually great and Ellie was so happy there. A few years later, I was worried again when Joey started preschool, because it can be different for boys than girls. When Joey was four years old, I went back to work part-time teaching in his preschool, which was really a gift because I could still be with him during the day and see how he was doing there. One of the parents once asked me, "How do I explain your family to my kids?" I was so glad she came to me with her question, and I said, "What we would ask is that you explain to your children that Ellie and Joey have two parents that really love them." That is how we choose to be in the world.*

*Both Ellie and Joey have the same donor so are biological siblings. When our kids were in elementary school I wondered if they thought about who their donor was. A dear friend of mine kindly relieved my mind by saying, "Callie, I don't think it is anywhere on their radar because they feel so loved by two parents. They don't long for anything more than what you and Lesley are giving them." For Ellie and Joey to grow up in these times, witnessing so many positive changes, including the acceptance of gay marriages, has been especially wonderful for our children.*

*Lesley and I both had moms who worked full time when we were growing up. My brother and I grew up in an in-home day care; we even went to the elementary school near our day care so we could go there after school rather than our neighborhood school. My mom and dad both needed to work when we were little. Lesley and I decided we didn't want that for our kids. My mom has even told our children that she feels badly she wasn't able to be with my brother and I after school and how fortunate they are to have had me at home. I do remember as a child, however, that when my mom got home from work, she'd put everything else aside and just spend that time with us kids reading, playing, and being involved with us. I know she probably stayed up late to get the dishes, housework, and laundry done, but she never did those things while we were awake. The connection I have with my mom, and had with my dad, has always been very close, because whenever I was present, they were present. This seems much more difficult for parents to maintain these days with the constant distraction of smart phones, but it's so important, especially when parents are separated all day from their kids.*

*We've explained to the kids, now that they're older, about the choices we've made in order to have more time with them and not be financially stressed as a family. When they were in elementary school I never missed a walk home with our kids at the end of a day. Lots of their friends' parents have beautiful large houses. When Ellie talks longingly about them, I always ask if she knows how much it would cost just for the electricity, water, home repairs, and the other workings of such a house. We emphasize to the kids that they should only buy what they can pay for. That is a value we live by* *and want our kids to understand how important it is. If they are five dollars short on a wish they have, then they either need to wait until next month's allowance or if they are interested in washing the car tomorrow, that is an option. This seems especially significant since I recently heard that the average American carries $13,000 in credit card debt, I don't want my kids to have that stress in their lives and relationships.*

*Lesley and I are a great match for each other and get along really well. We believe that a successful marriage comes from doing a lot of giving and compromising. I hear other women complaining that their husbands or partners don't help enough with the kids or housework, but it's important to have empathy for your partner and realize that each of you is adding to the family in a different way. Lesley and I both work hard contributing to our family and we do our best to acknowledge each other. It's just the little appreciations that mean so much. Lesley has always let me know how much she appreciates all that I do for the kids and I know it means a lot to her when I say, "Wow, you work so hard for us." I think it is good for our kids to hear us say these things to each other.*

*Something that I believe was very important in terms of keeping Lesley and my relationship close was that we always got the kids to bed early so we could spend the evening time together. Every night we made sure that we could sip a decaf and have our few hours to talk, share our days, and reconnect with each other. This was particularly important since we were living in such different worlds from each other during the daytime. Since Lesley and I were on such a tight budget, we couldn't afford to hire a babysitter and go out to a nice dinner. When we were honest with our friends and family about this, they offered to take care of the kids whenever we wanted a break. Something that has been really good for us as a couple is that we have allowed friends and family to give us those date nights. It is such a huge gift to offer a couple with young children an evening of childcare. Once you birth children, that connection is so intense; it took me some time to be able to leave the kids with anyone. It's important to trust that your kids will be okay if you leave them with family and friends who love them. When the kids were no longer little babies, we tried to carve out time as a couple to go have a quick inexpensive dinner together. It seemed a good way to help the kids to get used to being with other people who all have their own unique styles. I think that helping kids trust other people makes those first days of preschool, kindergarten, and all new experiences with others so much easier.*

*I sure hope that the tides will turn and the US will follow the European lead in terms of supporting new families. My cousins all live in Denmark and when they have their children they get an automatic six months of paid leave and then they can apply to have another six months of time off and they never have to worry about losing their jobs. The government realizes that the first year is actually the most critical year for mothers to be with their babies. Ellie recently said that when she grows up she wants to have a good job, but also wants to be a good mom. If she was living in Europe she could easily do both, but it is certainly harder in the US. I wish we would wake up as a country and realize that what we put in at the beginning will benefit our children for the rest of their lives in terms of their security, success in school, and relationships. Even if all American parents who possibly could, would stay home with their kids for even the first year, I believe that when those kids are older, they would be in much better shape than if they spent that first year away from a parent who loves and wants to be with them.*

*I worked as a teacher from the time Joey was in preschool until recently and am now home again being the caregiver to my own mom. After Mom was diagnosed with Parkinson's disease, we made a decision as a family that having time with Mom was what we wanted to be doing. Our commitment is that I will not get another job until Mom is no longer with us. It's so amazing to be able to help Mom through this stage of life and she is so grateful. I believe that if you nurture your babies, they will be able and willing to nurture you when you need it. It's been interesting to me how similar the nurturing of my elderly parent is to the nurturing I did with my babies in the first three years of their lives. I remember looking at my babies and having this feeling of awe that this being I love so much didn't exist in my life such a short time ago, and now I look at my mom who I've loved from the beginning of my life and I feel that same feeling of awe that in a short time she will no longer exist in this way. I feel that this time with Mom is so very special and I'm extremely thankful that I am not missing it, just like I felt with my babies.*

## Stay-at-Home Moms

*Nothing is more important to me than our girls . . .*
*Our first job is to make sure that our kids are on point.*
*That is the most important legacy we will ever leave.*
—Michelle Obama

An infant and mother are in a closely synchronized relationship, which began during the forty weeks of pregnancy and continues throughout the next forty weeks of complete dependency outside of the womb. When newborns feel the safety of a securely-attached, harmonious bond with their moms, they are able to relax and settle into breathing, sleeping, breastfeeding, digesting food, adapting to living in this world, and putting energy into growing a more sophisticated brain. The importance of the secure mother-infant dyad during this second half of gestation is understood around the world. This is the reason that babies are constantly worn on their mothers' bodies in developing countries and mothers are given at least a year of maternity leave in most developed countries.

Breastfeeding moms and babies bodies continue to be hormonally in sync; moms often awaken at night, feeling their breasts fill with milk even before their babies wake up hungry for their nighttime meal. So, it is no wonder that the majority of moms and tiny babies have much difficulty if they must be separated all day long when moms need to return to work. Moms that are able to stay at home longer can continue in a more natural intuitive rhythm with their babies. While being an at-home parent is a big change in a mom's life, most have no regrets later that they were able to spend this precious time with their baby.

A dad's care of the mom is a factor of greatest importance in terms of her having a positive pregnancy, birth, breastfeeding, and stay-at-home relationship with the baby. Being an at-home mom is an extremely demanding 24/7 job. Having the baby's dad give her some appreciation and champion what an important job she is doing can make a big difference in her feeling valued. This can also go a long way in boosting her overall contentment with caregiving the baby and satisfaction with their relationship as a couple. Dads in peaceful cultures understand that caring for new moms is the most valuable thing they can possibly do to help ensure their babies get the maternal nurturing they need. Dads who do a lot of holding, cuddling, bathing, rocking, singing, and dancing with their babies, when they finish breastfeeding and are ready to interact, really help at-home moms get a much needed break.

Stay-at-home moms additionally need support from extended family and other moms. During my year at home with my son, I remember looking out the window at 9:00 a.m. one morning and realizing that I was the only person in the neighborhood who was still there. I felt so out of touch with my colleagues and friends who were at work all day. There is a strong sense of loneliness that at-home moms feel, especially if they do not have other friends who are also home with babies. When I watched mothers in peaceful cultures gather in the village or at the river and heard them joyfully talking, laughing, and delighting in their children, it was clear that having such support kept those moms content at the most demanding job they would ever do. The only time I ever heard a Balinese mother speak angrily to her baby was when the young mother had left her village and was living in a big city isolated from others and with her husband gone all day. A lonely mom who doesn't have friends also dealing with the same life issues can become impatient, irritable, jealous, sad, guilty, or resentful, and then want to blame someone for her pain. Unfortunately, she often targets those she loves and needs the most. This is not a good equation for personal or marital satisfaction.

When I was doing my doctoral work as a psychologist, very little research had investigated the needs of a woman during her transition to motherhood. I decided to create some mother-infant support groups that met for ten structured weekly sessions and then were encouraged to continue meeting on their own. My findings were that being in a mothers' group resulted in greatly reduced feelings of isolation, positive feelings of support and camaraderie, more informed and relaxed attitudes toward mothering, a decrease in postpartum depression and anxiety, and increased marital satisfaction. My research led to some helpful start-up funding for a wonderful local group called Birth To Three created by some innovative women, that has provided parenting support to ninety-three thousand moms and dads over the past thirty-six years. When my daughter was born, thirty years ago, I joined a Birth To Three support group of older moms, and we formed such an important bond that the moms still meet a few times a year in what we now jokingly refer to as our Birth To Thirty group. Moms need other moms to remind each other that this stage of life, while stressful, is also uniquely precious and while the days seem long, the years fly by. You will never do a more important job, or feel as needed and loved by anyone ever again as you do by your infant or toddler. If there are not such organized groups available, consider asking moms from your prenatal swim, yoga, or birthing classes if they'd like to get together. You may need to reach past your comfort zone, but most likely the other moms are also longing for such contact and will be forever grateful that you took the first step.

Many stay-at-home moms worry that they won't ever be able to enter their career again if they stay home too long. I remember similar feelings as a young mom, and even though we don't have the job guarantees available in other countries, I certainly did not have trouble re-entering my profession, and am still working at it nearly forty years later.

## Stay-at-Home Mom Works From Home

*Valerie's Story:*

*I am a teacher of elementary-aged children and quit my job when I started trying to get pregnant, in order to have a more energetically healthy pregnancy for the baby. If there had been paid maternity leave in this country, I would have seriously considered not leaving my job, because I would have loved to have that job to come back to after a few years at home with the baby. But I knew I would not leave the baby at twelve weeks of age with someone else, so decided to go ahead and quit as I entered the childbearing stage of my life. During my pregnancy, even though I worked part-time doing some childcare, we still went into debt. In the grand scheme of things, I have no regret about quitting my job when I did, because it allowed me to have a much more relaxed pregnancy that felt like a gift to my gestating baby and myself.*

*After Ramona was born, I was delighted to be a mom and knew I didn't want to return to work anytime in the foreseeable future. We have been able to make ends meet by caring for the daughter of another new mom I met in a yoga class when we were both pregnant. When my friend Ashley needed to return to work, her baby daughter, Amy, six months old, began spending every workday in our home. It's fun for me to have "forty-hour-a-week twins," and it is easier than I expected taking care of two babies who are about the same age and developmental stage, liking the same toys, books, foods, activities, etc. Ramona, now a year old, loves our "Amy days," and the two toddlers have definitely become best buddies. This caregiving relationship is a dream come true. My husband, Jack, and I joke about how Amy feels like part of our family and that her parents feel like our extended family. I'm now thinking that I want to further extend my time as an at-home mom by caring for one or two more toddlers in the next few years. Hopefully taking care of other friends' children might feel like the extended family just continues to get bigger.*

*Jack has been very involved in Ramona's care and loves spending time with her. After I nurse her on a weekend morning, we'll trade off as to which of us gets up and lets the other parent have a few more hours of sleep. Jack is a teacher and during the school year he is gone for ten to twelve hours on weekdays. Not only is this a long time for me to be a solo parent, but also he misses having time with Ramona.*

*Jack, and I notice how much harder it is than the decade when we were together before being parents. We used to have our routines and household chores divided up quite comfortably, but having Ramona in our lives has certainly changed things! There seems to be twice as much work, but much less time, energy, or chance to get a break. It is difficult finding any time to just be together as a couple, and when we do, we're often too exhausted to really enjoy it. Jack and I feel closer to each other in terms of being a family unit, but often crave more time, attention, and just plain appreciation from the other about how hard each of us is working. It helps when I remind both of us that this stage in life is temporary; these may be the hard years for us as a couple, but they will pass. And we feel confident that the time we're putting in now is helping Ramona become the self-assured, compassionate, and happy toddler in whom we both are taking great delight.*

## Adoptive Parents with Stay-at-Home Mom

*Nancy and Roger's Story:*
(Attachment Deprived Child in Chapter 6 as told from parents' point of view.)

**Roger:** *We adopted two babies from China who are now nine and five years old. Julia came home with us when she was ten-months-old and four years later, Leonardo, thirteen-months-old, joined our family. We had waited until we were in our late thirties and financially secure before having children, because of not wanting to use day care when they were infants or toddlers. Our extended families live more than a thousand miles away, so even though we wish we could raise our children in a village, we can only rely on each other. We feel very fortunate to have careers that pay us well; we have not lived extravagantly, and never have large bills that need to be paid off. I was very glad the Federal Family Leave Act required my boss to give me three months off after each of the adoptions. I had saved up lots of paid vacation and sick leave so was able to get full pay during my paternal leaves. After Nancy and I had taken our twelve weeks of parental leave for Julia, Nancy was able to work part-time three or four mornings a week and I began working from 1:00 p.m. to midnight. On Nancy's workdays, I would take Julia to her mom's workplace about noon, and we'd switch cars because Julia had usually fallen asleep in the car seat. One of the hardest things for us as new parents was that we both felt very sleep deprived. I didn't get home until late, Nancy had a hard time getting to sleep in the evenings until I got home, and we both had to get up early in the morning for either work or Julia care.*

**Nancy:** *When Julia was adopted, she was very traumatized. In ten months, she had lost her birth mother, foster family, and was suddenly in a new country where absolutely nothing was familiar and was being cared for by parents who looked different and spoke a completely foreign language. For many months Julia would cry for seven hours a night as we tried walking, talking, dancing, reading, and everything else with her that we could possibly think of. We were getting desperate, but could not find* *any parenting books that helped us know what we could do to comfort our inconsolable child. The single most important breakthrough in terms of attachment was when I bought Julia into our bed at night. I realized that in order to build trust, Julia would need to feel that we were listening to her and respecting what she was trying to tell us. We finally understood that she could teach us how to be her parents, what we needed to do was watch and listen.*

*Once Julia began attaching to me, it was really hard when I left for work; there were even some days that I took a sick day and stayed home, because she was just too upset for me to leave her. In order to help Julia understand our daily schedules and not be so fearful of being abandoned again when either of us left, we did a lot of role-playing with a toy house, little people, and toy cars, showing her what that day or the next would be like. I paid attention to what seemed to bother Julia, and was always hunting for books with pictures that might help her understand her new world. We showed her books about being adopted, looking different from your parents, mommies and daddies going to work, trying to sleep at night (always an issue for her), and anything that seemed to provide some comfort. It really helped when we accepted that it was okay for her to be mad at us, and to this day listening to all of Julia's feelings, even the uncomfortable ones, is an important part of keeping our relationship close.*

*Something that was especially valuable starting when Julia was a baby was that we hired a college student who would come to the house for a few hours once a week and play with her. I would never leave, but was able to get a lot done around the house—such as paying bills and doing things that are hard to do with a baby wanting my attention.*

**Roger:** *Even though I resisted the co-sleeping at first, because of my upbringing, I really think it was most important in terms of Julia attaching to us. Nancy and I had tried taking turns being in Julia's room with her, even lying next to the crib all night, but that just didn't work. Julia wouldn't look at us, cried so much, and was just having a horrible time. It seemed like after only a week of sleeping in bed between us, she finally started attaching. She began looking at us, started smiling, and even laughed, all of which we hadn't experienced during the previous six months that she'd been with us.*

*I imagine just like most babies in the world, Julia had probably bed-shared and been worn on her foster mom's body, never having been alone, especially at night. We hadn't been exposed to such nurturing childrearing practices in our own traditional childhoods and had never considered how our ways must have felt to Julia.*

*When we began Leonardo's adoption, Nancy applied for a second maternity leave, but the next day her boss "let her go" due to downsizing. Nancy at that point became a stay-at-home mom and still is four years later. This meant I needed to be working full time, to provide the required income and health insurance. In retrospect, Nancy losing her job was probably a blessing in disguise because we didn't have to do so much "passing the baton" with Leonardo, and it just seemed easier for him to attach. He has been a lot more easy-going. I think it also helped that he had a sister who looked like him, and was quite nurturing with him. All three of us started co-sleeping with Leonardo from the very beginning, while we were still in China. Leonardo clearly attached first to his mom who was always with him and still prefers to be with her. I have felt left out at times in terms of my relationship with him, but also realize that everyone in our family has a job to do. While I may have drawn the short straw in terms of time with the kids, I am very glad the kids enjoy being with their mom. It has also created more flexibility for me to do lots of things that Nancy doesn't get to do. I've gotten more time to do hobbies and exercise, and appreciate that Nancy understands that I really need these outlets to unwind after working so many hours at my demanding and highly stressful job.*

*Some couples need two incomes just to get by if they're working at minimum wage jobs. But of the couples we know who have two professional incomes, there is definitely a shift happening toward wanting a parent at home with their babies and young children. In our life and our friends' lives, having time with families is once again becoming a high priority. Usually the mother is staying home and when she does go back to work only wants to work twenty to thirty hours per week as long as the other parent is working full time. We live in a society that values having a lot of material things and some people get hooked into thinking they absolutely have to have those things, so those parents will need to have two full-time incomes. Nancy and I value having a parent at home rather than more money and someone else raising our kids. We've definitely had to simplify our lifestyle to reduce our expenses. We don't eat out or go to movies any more. We don't take expensive trips like we used to do each year and instead we now go camping. We have decided not to buy the latest and greatest electronics and our sixteen-year-old car still runs just fine. Sure, we might get our dream car in twenty years, but for now, especially while the kids are young, we'd rather have more time with them.*

*Having kids has certainly changed our marital relationship. Some of the things that were really important before just no longer seem a priority. Nancy and I had been together over fifteen years before we had children, so we knew each other very well. There were many times, especially with our first baby, when Nancy was overly stressed and would get mad at me for seemingly no reason. I realized it was best at those times to bite my tongue and just take it, reminding myself, "this too shall pass."*

*Nancy: When we first brought Julia home, there was a period of time which was very hard on our marriage. I think we were both in shock, wondering what in the world we had done to our lives? I remember thinking that I just didn't know how to do this job, and I became incredibly overprotective of Julia. I would even protect her from how Roger was caring for her, and he's a great dad. I watched myself blaming him for things that he had no responsibility for; I don't know why I did that, the poor guy! If Julia fell on the other side of the room, I'd yell at Roger, "Why didn't you do something to keep her from falling?" We laugh at that now, but it was hard at the time. Roger did a good job of understanding that I was overwhelmed and scared; thankfully he didn't fight back. I think that after I got through my irrational new mom stage, I was able to come back to earth and realize I could do this mothering job and that everything was going to be okay.*

*One of the biggest things that switched for Roger and I was consciously deciding we are on the same team rather than rivals; this also helped us to have more empathy for each other. When I stop and try to imagine how things feel for Roger, to really put myself in his place, a new level of understanding begins to dissipate my anger. When Julia was little and I tried to imagine how it would feel to be at work until midnight with* the constant demands of Roger's highly responsible ten-hour job, when getting only four or five hours of sleep every night, this enabled me to have more compassion when he wanted to take a six-mile run before going back to another day of that. Roger and I have also created a few important ground rules for our family that have certainly helped. We try to really listen to each other (seek to understand, before you seek to be understood), talk to each other with respect, and not do any name-calling when we are angry. At first Roger and I would need to remind each other of these rules by saying, "Talk to me like I'm someone you love." Now this has simply become a much-appreciated habit. It also helps when we tell each other specifically what we need rather than believing we can read each other's mind. For example, I will say, Roger, I need two hours this weekend to get some sewing done. That way he's not guessing at what I need. While obviously neither of us gets everything we want, we do our best to take care of each other.

**Roger:** Ultimately, my relationship with Nancy has gotten much better. Prior to having children we were both used to focusing on our own desires and were pretty self-absorbed. After having children, our free time went from being fairly plentiful to being extremely scarce. It definitely took time for us both to adjust to the roles we had chosen and there were occasions in which Nancy didn't feel respected for the hard job she was doing as the parent at home. When Nancy complained about how difficult her job was, I tried to be supportive, but would sometimes feel resentful because my own job felt so stressful. A few times I made comments that I shouldn't have, like, "I'd trade places with you any day," and as would be expected, that went very poorly. I'm terrible at giving positive reinforcement. I usually tell people that if I say nothing, then just assume you are doing great—but that doesn't work very well at home. Nancy clearly wanted some appreciation. This for me is a work in progress, I'm doing better, but I'm certainly not sitting in the front of the class, yet. I still sometimes feel jealous of the time Nancy has with the kids, but I'm actually glad this is how it worked out.

**Nancy:** For me, being the parent stuck in the house all day would sometimes really get to me. I'm constantly busy trying to meet both kids' needs.

*It was hard for me when I complained to Roger about this and felt my job stress being minimized when he said something like, "count your blessings," or "you're lucky to be at home." When Roger comes home and the house isn't clean, I just don't care; it may not be clean until Leonardo is in third grade! We had a period when we weren't communicating well about any of this; I didn't feel valued in the job I was doing as a mother. It helped when Roger was able to explain to me that he wasn't devaluing the job I was doing, it was more about his own dissatisfaction with the stress he was feeling at his own job. I realized that I just needed to let it go, and accept that we were both working extremely hard and doing our best. Sometimes I would tell Roger that I needed an apology and he would usually apologize. When I'd ask, "Did you really mean that?" and, when he answered, "Yes, I did, I love you very much," it just made everything okay again.*

*Neither of our kids has ever been in day care, but we started each of them in a half-day preschool after they were three and a half years old. They were ready by then for that type of learning experience and enjoyed the socialization with other children. Roger and I don't have time alone together like we used to have, but we try to make the most of the time we do have to help us unwind and reconnect. We've even recently started taking a jujitsu class together, completely out of the realm of something we've ever previously considered, and it's been a great way to get rid of pent-up tensions. We also try to use a lot of humor to get through difficult times and try not taking things too seriously—Roger is especially good at that! He usually gets us laughing, often at ourselves, and that really makes things more positive for all of us.*

**Roger:** *Some friends who have delightful, productive older children once told us, "you need to put a certain amount of effort into helping each child be successful; if you put it in early, your life will be much easier later on. But if you wait until they are teenagers, then things will be much more difficult and it may be too late." Nancy and I want to have kids we enjoy being around, so we took our friends' advice and decided to put the time in now. We feel very fortunate to have been able to have a parent at home and realize the benefit for our children of doing it this way.*

## Stay-at-Home Dads

*When I look at the relative importance of what life is about,*
*I can't quite convince myself that making a record*
*Or having a career is more important,*
*Or even as important, as my child, or any child.*

—John Lennon

Current generation dads who talk to their babies while in utero, are closely involved in the births, cut the baby's cord, and hold their tiny newborns skin-to-skin in the hour after birth, are experiencing elevated levels of hormones that promote attachment, caregiving, and protection of their wives and babies. Like fathers in the peaceful cultures, Gen Y dads in the US are taking over the household chores, cooking meals, and spending the first few weeks after the birth caring for the mother and baby, while forming their own close attachment during this period of family bonding. Hands-on fathers are becoming more nurturing and are often caring for all the infant's needs except for breastfeeding.

When today's parents are deciding who will take care of the newborn after the maternity leave, some are choosing for the mom to be the working parent and the dad to be the at-home parent. Although American women still on average earn only seventy-eight cents for every one-dollar that a man earns, there are many mothers who have higher paying jobs with better benefits than their baby's father, or sometimes the dads are unemployed. Deciding who will be the at-home parent should not be based on income alone, however, because the importance of a mom being home to comfort-nurse and feed the baby during the first year cannot be discounted. In most developing countries, the mother will be the at-home parent until the baby is old enough to be eating solid foods and then the dad will share the next few years of being at home until the three-year-old enters preschool. Many couples in the US are making similar decisions, but since we don't have parental leave options supported by the government, parents must take into account each family member's individual needs along with career and financial responsibilities, creating a solution that works best for all family members. An extremely important consideration are the personalities of the parents: the one who is the most nurturing, patient, and truly enjoys babies will most likely make the best at-home parent. Although a stay-at-home dad is a relatively new phenomenon, there are currently two million fathers in the US who are the primary caregivers of their children, with twenty percent of fathers being the at-home parent when the child's mom is employed.[3]

As mentioned in the section about stay-at-home moms, being a stay-at-home parent is a tremendously challenging and isolating job. Stay-at-home dads deserve much emotional support and appreciation from the working mom, which will certainly help dad feel respected and increase the overall happiness of the couple and family. It is also important for the stay-at-home parent to offer the working parent special recognition, such as one happily married couple I've worked with in which the at-home dad makes a point of greeting his wife at the end of the workday with such words as, "Hey kids, here's that mommy of yours who works so hard for us!"

Although stay-at-home dads might not have the same deep need to talk about their parenting feelings and issues as much as moms, it still helps when they have the support of other parents and at least one other stay-at-home dad with whom to spend time. Many dads feel that being the at-home parent for some part of their children's early years was the most rewarding career choice they ever made.

## Stay-at-Home Dad from Infancy to Age Five

*Sam's Story:*

*When Buffy found out she was pregnant it was quite a surprise. We were living together, but not married. She had a great job working as a business executive and I was working as a caregiver. I loved my job and it had great health benefits, but I was only making a bit over minimum wage. If I'd continued working after the baby was born, my entire salary would have gone to pay someone else to raise our kid, which just didn't make sense to either of us. We decided that with Buffy's salary, we wouldn't be rich, but could afford to have me at home with the baby. After she was pregnant, that decision came pretty quickly and easily; it just made sense. So, we put a down payment on a house, and started putting some money aside to use after the baby was born.*

*My attachment to Baby Alice began during the pregnancy. When Buffy was about six or seven months along, there was a guy who was ready to step into my job, so I stopped working. That gave me a couple of months before Alice was born to get the new house fixed up, prepare things, and I did a lot of the nesting.*

*Buffy planned to take three months of unpaid leave after Alice was born, but she started working some after about two and a half months. For those first ten weeks, it was so awesome! We'd just had this baby, it was just the three of us, and we just hung out together. We walked and hiked some with Alice and watched her eat and sleep. It was such a great time! Buffy still talks about how special it was for her. Then Buffy started working a bit from home, going to meetings, and by three months she was back at the office full time. Her job was really supportive of her time at home with the baby. When Alice was six months old, Buffy and I got married.*

*After Buffy went back to work, she was still breastfeeding for about a year and would leave pumped breast milk in the freezer. But every day I would drive over to the office so Alice could nurse from her mom rather than have Buffy pumping milk while at work. I'd go once a day for sure around Buffy's lunch break and sometimes I'd go again later in the day. Then Buffy would come home at night and breastfeed Alice. We planned to do this for two years, but at about a year old, when I'd take Alice to the office, she was more interested in looking around, biting at the breast, and playing. Alice clearly let us know that she was finished with nursing.*

*For me it has been really good being an at-home dad. I'm definitely a nurturer and being a caregiver comes naturally for me. I am a good listener, very attentive, like to play, and as a musician I enjoy playing music with Alice. I also have a lot of patience, which certainly has been tested many, many times by being with a child all day, every day. As Alice got older, there were definitely times that I'd tell her I needed a break and she needed to go play by herself. Alice is five years old now and I've been doing this job for her entire life. I do most of the housework, cleaning, laundry, yard work and car repair. I'm not a good cook and Buffy loves to cook, so she shops for food and makes most of our dinners.*

*This role reversal was actually hardest for Buffy at first. When she told people she was working and I was the stay-at-home parent, they'd just assume it was because of the economy that I couldn't get a job. When Buffy told them that we had chosen for me to be the one at home, they seemed really surprised. It is hard on Buffy to be gone from Alice all day. There are definitely times when I'm telling her about our day that I can tell she feels sad to be missing out. But although Buffy likes having weekends just with Alice when I'm out of town, she doesn't have the depth of patience that I do. I tend to be more the family nurturer, maybe it's just because I'm used to being the at-home parent or because I'm a caregiver. But Buffy and Alice definitely have a special bond from pregnancy and breastfeeding, and when Alice gets hurt or wants someone to cuddle her, she always goes to her mom. When Buffy gets home after work, she and Alice reconnect by reading books, snuggling a lot, talking, and cooking together. On weekends they love to take long naps snuggled up with each other. Buffy and I were aware it wasn't traditional for me to be the stay-at-home parent and for her to be working, but it just seemed natural for us and it has worked well. It has not only been best for us financially, but also for both of our personalities.*

*Being a very social person really helps a great deal. With only one child, I'm able to get out and it's easy for me to connect with people who have kids and those who don't. When I was first at home with Alice, I'd wear her in a front pack and walk around town and go to the library for story time, or to the park. I live in a very open-minded liberal community so I usually felt pretty much accepted. Every so often, however, when I walked up to a group of moms and tried to pseudo join the conversation, I'd get a quizzical "who's this guy" feeling from them. Like they had to sorta protect their children from me. I felt that if I was a woman, they would have been more open with me. But when other stay-at-home mom friends of mine arrived and I'd be playing with their kids and the other moms realized I was a stay-at-home dad, they seemed more accepting. We now have a big network of friends who share parenting with us, and since Alice has gotten older she goes and plays at others' houses when I have something else I need or want to do. We have no extended family in town, which I think would be awesome, but we have created a big network of people who are part of "our village."*

*It took a few years before I met another stay-at-home dad who became a good friend. His son and Alice are the same age and he has a daughter who is two years younger. His wife is a doctor; she works and he stays home. It's been good to hang out with him, our kids like to play together, and our families have become close. He doesn't talk about getting much flak for being a stay-at-home dad, and it's clearly his gig. When we're together, playing with the kids, like while throwing a Frisbee, we definitely talk some about our kids and our feelings about parenting, but most the time we typically talk about other things. This has been great for me, because when I'm with a group of moms, I find that the conversation is constantly about parenting and the kids; it sometimes just gets too much for me. I used to believe that there were no differences between men and women; it is just how we are raised. But now that I've gone through all this, I definitely know that there are big, distinct differences between boys and girls, and men and women in terms of their basic instincts, how they react to things, and what they find is important.*

*I absolutely believe that dads are becoming more nurturing. There are a lot more instances of dads coming home from work and the first thing they want to do is spend time with their kids. I think this is much more prevalent than in past generations. I'm sure that there are guys out there who don't value nurturing, but I just don't encounter them. There's that stereotype of male macho behavior and I think it probably exists, but even with young guys, I don't see that in any of them. I can't even imagine someone saying, "Oh you stay at home with your kid, what a wimp." I think there is really a societal change happening. Perhaps it's from TV, or the Internet, I don't know, but even back home in my small conservative mid-west town, I have yet to run across that machismo attitude toward being a father.*

*My best friend is a teacher, his wife works part-time and has been the primary caregiver of their two kids. He's told me that if he had his way, they'd both work half-time and each spend the other half with the kids. He's jealous that I get to be a stay-at-home dad. He loves the summertime when his entire focus can be on spending time with his kids. They get chores done in the morning and then they hang out playing or doing fun things together for the rest of the day and go camping whenever they want.*

*A lot of parents are realizing that our kids are small for such a short amount of time. Parents don't get enough time to just be with their kids* when working full time and are often too tired when they get home to really enjoy them. But I have also talked to dads and moms who, although they love their kids, clearly prefer to go to work. I think it takes special nurturing energy to enjoy being with kids all day, and if you don't have that, it would probably feel like torture. One of the biggest problems for parents today is the need to limit the constant distraction of our cell phones and tablets. It's so hard to focus on being with your kids when there is that continual disturbance. Buffy and I don't allow media interference during our dinner times. I've even had to tell my parents to put their phones away at the table.

Buffy and I sometimes have date-nights, but we don't do it very much because it is too expensive. Since having one income, we've definitely cut back on expenses by not going out, not taking many vacations, and biking rather than driving a car whenever we can. Since Alice was two-and-a -half years old, she's loved spending the night with some of our close network of friends. When Alice has a sleep over, Buffy and I definitely like to go out and do things together. Trading overnights with other parents has really helped us get some special time together without costing too much.

There are a few things that have been really stressful on our marriage. The hardest is that Buffy needs to travel for her job and is gone for a few days a couple of times a month. Although it's stressful for all of us when Buffy is gone, Alice and I get a good routine going and it's always difficult when Buffy gets back home. Buffy's reentry with us is really hard, we've all been having such different experiences and it's hard to find a way to reconnect. Another stressful thing for us as a couple are those times when Buffy is overworked and stressed about some deadlines at work, but I need her to come home. I'm in theater and sometimes need to go to play rehearsals, which even though unpaid are really important to me. There may be a month when I'm rehearsing every night, and Buffy comes home tired. We have dinner and then I'm gone until late at night. And when the show opens I'm gone every weekend night for many weeks. So, after working every day, Buffy needs to be home with Alice and doesn't have any time to do anything on her own for a couple of months. Those times are extra stressful, and when we have the most arguments.

Even though Buffy and I weren't sure we wanted to have children, and having a child has completely changed everything, having Alice has been the best decision in our entire lives. The greatest thing about being a stay-at-home dad has been watching Alice grow up and being able to influence her life, and she certainly has influenced mine. I feel very lucky to have been able to be an at-home parent, and know lots of families who just can't afford to have one of the parents stay home.

My dad was in the air force and my mom was always at home taking care of my older brother and I when we were young. Even though my mom had a degree in library science and had liked working in that job, as an air force officer's wife she was discouraged from having a career. I'm glad I had my mom at home and didn't grow up in day care, and I didn't want that for Alice. Even if I'd had a six-figure job, I just wouldn't have wanted someone else to raise my kid. My military family moved around a lot and never lived near any extended family. But now I am trying to talk my retired parents along with my brother and his wife into moving out here because I'm realizing how wonderful it would be to have family in town. I wasn't raised with that, but I'd love to have that for Alice. My parents are older and wouldn't be able to be hands-on caregivers since they really can't keep up with a five-year-old's energy. But if they could take care of her even one night a month, that would be amazing! I have friends whose own parents are the primary caregivers when the parents are at work, and I would be so fine with providing that for Alice someday if I'm a grandparent.

When Alice was three years old, she started preschool two mornings a week. At four, she went three mornings, and now at five, she'll be going four mornings a week for four and a half hours. So, I now have eighteen hours a week available to do other things. I'm beginning to do some caregiving, theater camps for kids, and odd jobs while Alice is at preschool. I've loved being a stay-at-home dad, but now it's time for me to start getting back out there and begin to make some money again.

## Unmarried Dad Stays Home for a Year with Toddler

*Alexander's Story:*

April and I were dating when we discovered she was pregnant. Even though we were unsure of whether we could make a long-term commitment to each other, we both made a lifelong commitment to our unborn baby. Since Scarlet's birth, I have delighted in being involved in her caregiving and even have lived most of the time in the same house with April and Scarlet to assure that I could help with finances, cooking, household chores, and care for the baby while developing my own strong attachment to my daughter. It was important to me to be an equally competent parent, comfortable with changing diapers, dressing, soothing, putting Scarlet down to sleep, and generally letting April know that she wasn't expected to do it all without my help. As a dad, I felt it was already unfair to April in terms of the responsibility she had taken on. I didn't carry the baby, give birth, couldn't breastfeed; there are a lot of things between the mom and baby that I just couldn't be a part of, so I tried to do everything else that I could do.

April and I had a month off together after the birth. It was great for us in terms of attaching to Scarlet; together we learned how to care for her at the same time. April then took another six weeks off before starting back to work. I wish at that point I'd had another month of paid leave so Scarlet could have still been cared for by one of her parents. I think the first six months can be tougher on a dad in terms of attachment. From the beginning minutes after the birth, mom is usually the first one who holds, soothes, and feeds the baby. From that moment on, the mom takes on the primary role and the baby wants to be with the mom. I think I was pretty good at soothing and comforting Scarlet and she would fall asleep in my arms, but I didn't have the experience of being pregnant or giving birth and didn't have the same hormonal attachment that April seemed to have. I think my attachment grew stronger when Scarlet was about six to nine months old, became more aware of me and started to seek me out, when she'd look at me and actually crawl over to me. I guess it was essentially when she started to clearly attach to me that I started to feel what that type of bond was really like.

I have heard that dads can feel jealous of the relationship the mom and baby have, but I certainly didn't feel that way at all and have never heard any of my dad friends mention feeling that way. I just felt it was really important that April succeed in having a close bond and good, strong breastfeeding experience with Scarlet, and was happy that the baby seemed to be very healthy and content. I think a mom has such an important role during those first months and I was glad April was doing such good job at meeting Scarlet's needs. April was able to exclusively breastfeed Scarlet for the first six months. Then April had to travel on a work trip and was gone for a few days. I burned through all the breast milk and had to use some formula. When April returned she began having problems producing enough breast milk, so we transitioned to foods and formula at that point.

I was pretty much working full time and although April was able to do most of her job by telecommuting from home, it was hard for her to get much work done when Scarlet was with her. Since we live in a country without any paid parental leave, we would have probably needed to use day care if we hadn't had family support, especially during that first year. April and I both felt strongly that we didn't want Scarlet to be in a strange place, bonding with people who wouldn't be part of her life later, rather than family members who would always be in her life. Having both sets of grandparents living in town has really made it possible for Scarlet to always be cared for by a family member. As soon as April had told her mom about the pregnancy, Grandma's first response was that she would be willing to care for the baby during the day when we were working. True to her word, Grandma has been very involved in Scarlet's life and is willing to watch her whenever we need help. From the time Scarlet was about ten weeks old she began spending a lot of time in April's parents' home. I would drop Scarlet off at Grandma's house on my way to work and she'd be picked up by April in the mid-afternoon, whenever she'd finished her work for the day. So Scarlet would usually spend five or six hours a day with Grandma. My mom was also willing to care for Scarlet whenever we needed extra help. I have always felt great about Scarlet being with her grandparents because I trust them all and I like the fact that they were getting time to bond with her. With all I've learned about the importance of early attachment and security building in my college child development classes and my job working with kids, I was very glad that loving grandparents were Scarlet's caregivers. Of course, it also has been so much better financially than using day care. It's just been a great scenario all around.

Although I went into the job of being a dad with a pretty good awareness that having a baby in my life would be a lot of work, I think the hardest thing for me initially was having no downtime for myself at all. Being a working dad, I would come home tired after a full day at my job and immediately be on baby duty. April often would already be stressed from doing her job and *having just spent the last few hours caring for Scarlet. As soon as I walked in the door, she'd hand me the baby saying, "Now it's your turn." The time demands especially with two working parents was difficult to manage. In the evening when I wanted to just relax a bit and decompress from the day, there was dinner to be made, a mess to clean up, and a baby that needed care. It was tough as parents to be happy and not just feel overly stressed.*

*When I was growing up I think we were the first generation of children that really didn't have grandparents, extended family, or often intact nuclear families in our lives. A lot of our parents had moved far away from their families. In the 1980s and 90s there were lots of divorces and uninvolved fathers. My dad was pretty absent from the time I was three; my parents divorced when I was about five and I only saw him a couple of weekends a month. I think when there is a split in a family, it has far reaching impact; it impacts the finances, the other parent, the children, how the siblings relate to each other, and just about everything. My mother was a busy single working mom of three children who was very financially stressed and had to work long hours including some night shifts. I'm sure she would have been a much happier mom if she hadn't been so strapped. I went to day care, then preschool, and we had a lot of different babysitters. We lived thousands of miles away from my grandparents and we never had any kind of extended family support whatsoever. I think there were lots of kids my age who had similar childhoods in which the focus on the family really went off track. One of the ways this seems to have influenced me and lots of young parents my age is that we want to do it very differently. We remember how impactful it was either not to have dads around or not to have very good relationships with them.*

*My generation tends to have high standards for what kind of parents we want to be and what kind of families we want to have. I have many friends in their early thirties who have decided not to even have children because they don't think they can provide the kind of experience that kids should have. My male friends who do have children, for the most part, are dads who want to be very involved in their kids' lives. For my generation, I think the idea of a dad not being involved from the beginning with their babies is just not even an option. My friends who are dads are definitely equal partners in parenting their children in all ways including nurturing, disciplining, and doing everything that they can, and they all have really good relationships with their kids. I believe that in order for humans to be strong and thriving and happy and healthy, it is most important to have happy, strong, and healthy families.*

*Scarlet is now two and a half years old and for the past year I have pretty much spent all of my time with her. After my department was downsized and I was suddenly without a job, I chose to become a stay-at-home dad. I decided that if a really good job came up I would take it, but otherwise I would opt to be the primary parent at home. April was making okay money working full time and I wanted to have that early toddler time with Scarlet. Even though there have been some financial stresses and I didn't know how long I would be without a job, originally thinking it might be just a few months, I have really enjoyed spending this entire year with my daughter. Scarlet has pretty much stopped going to grandma's house unless April and I take a special weekend together out of town. Being able to be the primary parent so much of the time has been a great experience. I take Scarlet out to the park, feed her lunch, put her down for a nap, give her a bath, and have become her number one playmate. I've learned that three of the most important things about being a good parent is delighting in your child, having patience, and being flexible (I really try to understand what she is wanting to do and ask myself whether there's a good reason for keeping her from doing that, rather than just sticking to a rigid predetermined plan). It is so great when parents can share in their children's world, have fun, and enjoy them. Being a parent has times when it is such hard work, so stressful, and exhausting. You definitely need those joyful times to balance it all out. I think the physical connecting part is also important, when Scarlet sits on my lap I'll stroke her hair, and she loves it when we dance together or sit next to each other watching a movie. I think the time I have spent with Scarlet is going to pay dividends with the two of us having a strong relationship for the rest of our lives.*

*April and I are still not married, but what has kept us together is that we are both so involved with Scarlet and she has such a strong relationship with each of us. We have always been focused on the goal of doing what was best for Scarlet. We sorta did it backward; we definitely became a family before we became a couple. I feel like being a couple is almost a new work in progress and there are still a lot of things that need to be worked out before I can make the commitment to get married or have any other children together. It seems to me like I need time to see April as a partner rather than only a co-parent; we are now beginning to work on building that type of intimacy.*

## Grandparents as Primary Caregivers

*I am happy to say all of my grandchildren are kind.*
*It's very important to me that people are kind.*
*I must be kind to myself first.*

—Maya Angelou

Traditionally around the world and even in this country during previous generations, grandmothers were automatically expected and delighted to be primary caregivers of their grandchildren. People valued having their extended families in their lives and cousins often grew up spending as much time together as siblings. In Japan, it is common for a maternal grandmother to quit her job when her daughter has the first grandchild so she can help her daughter be a successful mother. Many Japanese grandmothers move into their daughters' homes to help care for the new moms and babies while leaving grandfathers to be on their own for awhile as grandmothers embrace this new role in their lives.

During the Baby Boom Generation in the US, the majority of successful, young independent adults, (more likely insecurely attached due to the birthing and childrearing practices of the day), left their families of origin behind and moved to wherever the best educational or career opportunities were offered, often thousands of miles away. Jobs and money became much higher priorities than relationships with extended family members. Grandchildren of that generation were lucky to see their grandparents once or twice a year and certainly did not create close, intimate relationships with them. Most grandparents prided themselves on being free to spend their retired time focused on their own desires, with golfing, traveling, and RVing becoming the sought after norms, certainly not hands-on caregiving of grandchildren.

Today's Gen Y parents, who grew up without extended families remember longing for relationships with their grandparents and wondering what it would be like to have aunts, uncles, and cousins in their daily lives. Many young adults of this generation are trying to reconnect the lost support from families by returning "home" after college and/or inviting their parents and siblings to once again share in their lives. Most of the grandparents that I know seem delighted by this current social trend that is taking us back to the way things used to be when we had close secure attachments among family members. Humans throughout history have lived in multigenerational clans or tribes; we are not animals that are meant to live in isolation or tiny family groups, and are usually much healthier and happier when we have closely connected, loving relationships. In fact, the Bhutanese believe that the most important factor in terms of human happiness is to live near to your extended family.

An important factor that is influencing many of today's grandmothers to become more involved in their grandbabies' lives is that they were the first generation of mothers in this country that missed out on being at home with their babies due to the cultural changes that took place at that time. In an interview, American broadcast journalist Barbara Walters lamented, "I was so busy with a career. . . . And you know, on your deathbed, are you going to say, 'I wish I spent more time in the office?' No, you'll say, 'I wish I spent more time with my family,' and I do feel that way. I wish I had spent more time with my Jackie."[4] Grandchildren are giving these women another opportunity to be primary caregivers of babies and most are excited to have this second chance. It also helps that Boomer Gen women are tending to be healthier and live longer than previous generations with an average life expectancy of eighty-one years, a twenty-five year increase in over the past century. The cover story of a recent newsletter published by the American Association of Retired Persons (AARP) focuses on "The New Grandmothers," offering insight into creative ways that women are embracing the role of grandmother. Letty Cottin Pogrebin, cofounder of *Ms.* magazine and author of *Getting Over Getting Older,* remembers her grandmother "as a remote figure who spent all of her time cooking, cleaning, and taking care of others." In contrast, Pogrebin loves playing on the floor with her grandchildren, or canoeing with them across a lake, and telling them about her life and worldview.[5] Actress and author Jane Seymour delights in having two of her four grandchildren living nearby and spending two days a week caring for them. "My favorite days are when they come over—there's so much I want to give them, so much to share . . . It's a whole new form of love."[6] Although eighty percent of grandparents have some grandchildren living more than fifty miles away, they are taking advantage of modern technology to stay connected through digital methods such as texting, Skyping, Facebook, Face Time, Instagram, and by traveling by trains or airplane to visit them. Grandmothers of the boomer generation have a renewed dedication to be involved in their grandchildren's lives no matter what it takes.[7] Today's grandmothers are loving the close primary attachments they have with their grandchildren, which in many cases is also giving them the closer relationships with their sons and daughters that they missed during their own much-too-busy years of being working moms.

Programs such as Planet Grandparent and the GaGa Sisterhood offer workshops and support groups to help understand grandparenting challenges and become successful in this role. Their goals include involving grandparents as a positive force in their children's families by helping with caregiving, reducing maternal stress, sharing wisdom, providing grandchildren with unconditional love and generational history, promoting understanding with their adult children, and enhancing support for the entire family. Planet Grandparent also helps grandparents learn about modern relational childrearing practices and how they can be involved, but not intrusive, by honoring their own sons' and daughters' roles as the parents.[8]

Returning to a trend of previous generations, "multigen" living situations are taking place in which more than one generation is residing in the same home. A Pew Research Center analysis of the most recent US Census Bureau data indicates that approximately fifty-one million Americans, nearly seventeen percent of the population, are now living with at least two generations of related adults under-one-roof. This often includes a grandparent living with their son's or daughter's family. There was a ten and a half percent increase in multigenerational households from 2007 to 2009, and a 2012 survey done by a national home building group found that thirty-two percent of young adults expect to eventually be sharing a house with one of their parents. Some builders have even begun to offer homes with two master bedroom suites, or "Next Gen" homes consisting of one large house and an attached smaller one that can be adjoined by an inner door that when closed creates two separate living spaces. While this trend began during the tanked economy, it appears to be continuing and gaining momentum, with eighty-two percent of those who shared housing feeling that it brought them closer as a family, seventy-two percent welcoming the improvement in their finances, and seventy-five percent appreciating the benefits of being able to have built-in child and elder care.[9] Modern parents are moving from the quest for independence of the previous generation to valuing the interdependence seen in peaceful cultures that involve sharing chores, food preparation, expenses, and caring for grandchildren while the parents are working. The job of elders throughout evolution has always been to reach out to the younger generations and help mentor those grandchildren toward adulthood.

## Working Parents Using Grandmother and Friend

*Maria's Story:*

*My husband and I are both from other countries and do not have extended family living nearby. In my country I would have gotten three years of maternity leave with the first year paid by the government. Since there is no paid maternity leave in this country, after I got pregnant I asked my mom if she would come to the US for six months and help us care for the baby when I had to return to work. She actually loved the idea. After our baby, Sophia, was born, my employee short-term disability insurance paid seven of my twelve weeks of leave at seventy percent, which really helped us meet our expenses. But three months is too short a time to have with your baby; I wish I could have had the first year at home with her. Then I would have probably wanted to return to the career that I love. I don't think I have the personality to be a stay-at-home mom for too long, but I knew that I didn't want Sophia to be in a large day care where babies don't get enough nurturing from a loving caregiver. I heard about a day care where there were eight babies six weeks to six months old with strict policies such as babies could only be fed formula (no breast milk) every three hours, diapers changed every two hours, and day care workers weren't allowed to spend time rocking the babies to sleep. I knew that was not happening for my baby girl.*

*When Sophia was ten weeks old my mom came, stayed with us for six months, and took care of Sophia while I was at work. Before Grandma had to return home, I was lucky enough to discover that a stay-at-home mom friend, Mara, with a baby close to Sophia's age was willing to take care of my baby so Mara could stay home longer with her daughter. We started taking Sophia over there part-time when she was about seven months old, and by eight-and-a-half months she had fully transitioned to spending every week-day from early morning when I'd drop her off until her dad, Stephan, picked her up at the end of the day, which totaled about forty-five hours a week.*

*I met Mara in our birthing class when we were both pregnant. The women from that birthing class have continued meeting and a wonderfully supportive moms group has developed. We met weekly after our babies were born until most of the moms had to return to work, now we still meet when we can and even recently did a summer camping trip with all the dads and babies. In the past few months, Stephan and I even decided to move across town so we can be closer to two of the families in that group, including Mara's. The mom's group and living in this neighborhood has really helped me feel like I am part of a supportive village. I feel so comfortable leaving Sophia with Mara, whom I totally trust since we share the same childrearing and caregiving attitudes. Sophia has become very attached to Mara and her daughter and is absolutely happy to spend her days with them.*

*My parents are now retired and want to come to the US every year and spend a few months caring for Sophia. I think we'll still have her spend one day a week with Mara, to keep that relationship strong, because when my parents return home, Sophia will go back there full-time again.*

*I'm still breastfeeding Sophia who is now thirteen months old, and pump while at work. My workplace is extremely supportive and has provided a maternity lounge with comfortable chairs, music, and a refrigerator. The only problem is how much time it takes out of my day, which is close to an hour by the time I go to the lounge twice a day, set things up, and pump for about twenty minutes. At times there have been all day meetings and I've needed to pump discreetly in the back corner of the room and am thankful that everyone seems to be okay with that. I'd like to go down to pumping only once during the day, but Sophia is still drinking two full bottles each day, so I know she needs that much milk.*

*Stephan is very willing to help with Sophia by changing diapers and giving her a bath, but since I'm still nursing I usually put her to sleep. A lot of times when he tries to comfort her, she just wants me if I'm in the house and she will cry harder until I come, which makes him feel badly. But he's the one who can get her to take her daytime naps easier, by giving her a binky and rocking her to sleep. He picks her up from Mara's every evening and they have a few hours of daddy-daughter time before I get home from work. And, on the weekends, Stephan usually gets up with Sophia in the morning; they enjoy playing together for a few hours while I happily get some extra sleep.*

## Caregiving Grandma in Retirement Home

*Sophie's Story:*

*Before my husband and I even tried to get pregnant, we knew day care wasn't an option financially because we needed both of our salaries just to cover our expenses. There wouldn't be enough money left over to pay for day care, primarily due to the mortgage on our house and additional expenses of three older stepchildren. So, we asked my mom whether she would be willing to be a primary caregiver if we were able to have a baby. Mom was planning to retire soon and eagerly agreed to move into an independent-living retirement facility five minutes from where we lived, so she could take care of the baby when we returned to work. We also planned ahead by saving up some paid leave and extra money, so we could stay home for as long as possible once we had a baby.*

*During the last month of pregnancy I was able to work from home, and after our baby, Olivia, was born, I was lucky enough to have four months of paid leave. My employer gives one month of paid leave for each year of employment (up to three months) and I had saved up another month of paid vacation leave. My husband, Kyle, got two weeks of paid leave and he took another month of unpaid leave so he could care for Olivia and I during those important first six weeks after the birth.*

*I never suffered from the sleep deprivation that many new moms experience because Kyle was there to help. I would go to bed early with Olivia and when she woke up for the day at 5:00 a.m., Kyle would get up and take care of her, bringing her to me if she needed to nurse. I would gratefully continue sleeping and when I awoke a few hours later, Kyle usually had breakfast ready for me. This time of early attachment with Olivia was especially important to Kyle because he hadn't gotten it with his older children during the one to two weeks he'd had off.*

*After my four months of paid leave, I was still so panicked about the idea of leaving Olivia all day long and having to pump so she'd only have breast milk, that I asked my employer if I could work from home for another two months. Thankfully, he agreed, and during those two months of telecommuting, I actually worked from my mom's home. That way Olivia was able to get used to being cared for by my mom while I was there to answer Grandma's questions and interpret Olivia's needs. We set up Grandma's place so it felt welcoming to Olivia and it actually became an unexpected joy for other members in the retirement home to have a baby there each day. Folks would gather in the communal areas when Grandma and Olivia were there and the talk became delightfully animated by memorable stories of wonderful and trying times they had with their own children and grandchildren. Now that Olivia is a toddler, she enjoys pushing some of the older folks around in their walkers, which, of course, totally amuses and enchants them. Grandma says that she is willing to continue taking care of Olivia every weekday for as long as she is physically able.*

*I have continued to breastfeed Olivia in the evenings and weekends, but now that she is fifteen months old I have just recently stopped pumping breast milk when I'm at work. It was so exhausting to be pumping during every break. I just never ever really got a break for that entire year. It was also weird at work to have the milk let-down feeling and hormones firing with no baby there. I was at least lucky enough to have my own office where I could look at photos of the baby that my mom sent me during the day on the computer, while pumping milk. Some moms I know have to pump in a bathroom stall or in their parked car.*

*We still co-sleep with Olivia on a small mattress next to our large one that is also on the floor. I think that cuddling up with her in the evenings and spending our nights close to her, especially after being apart all day long, is critically important to help us reconnect and has absolutely made a difference in our relationship.*

*I was completely unprepared for how stressful having a baby would be on my marriage. I was so tired and my "mom brain" had such a singular focus on just caring about what happened with the baby that it was really hard to pay attention to anything else, including my husband. When we were both back working and then would come home, make dinner, do chores, spend time with the baby, and try to get some sleep, it was so hard to find any time to be together. It killed our sex life, and the only thing that worked for us was to schedule sex on certain nights of the week. Once we started to do that our entire relationship turned around. I still find it frustrating to schedule sex, but it keeps my husband happier and that is definitely better for all of us. I found out later that during the first year after the baby was born, my husband was really worried about whether our marriage would survive. I had never realized that he was taking some of our fights to such an extreme level of anxiety. We are now both taking a half-day off work during the week to go have a meal and spend some relaxed time with each other. Time to just enjoy being together the way we used to be has helped us feel much closer again.*

## Nanny as Primary Caregiver

*The things that matter most in our lives are not fantastic or grand.*
*They are the moments when we touch one another.*

—Jack Kornfield

"Nanny" refers to someone who cares for youngsters in the children's own home. The term's first known use was in 1795 and its origin is believed to have been baby talk for a loved caregiver. If neither of the parents, grandparents, or an attached family member is able to stay home and care for an infant or toddler, having a nanny is the next best option. When a baby can stay in his own familiar surroundings and not have to be gotten up, dressed, and taken to another place early each morning, there is usually much less stress for the child and the parents. Having a nanny allows a baby to have a consistent caregiver with whom he can form a closely connected, trusting relationship that hopefully will blossom into a love for each other. Of most importance is that the nanny be someone who is kind, responsive, nurturing, loves babies, and intends to care for the baby long-term, at best throughout the toddler years. All of us, especially babies, are hurt when we are in love with someone and that person suddenly leaves us. Each time this happens it takes us longer to trust again, and after too many losses we protect our hearts by becoming more guarded in relationships. As a psychologist, I most commonly saw this type of attachment disorder in children who had grown up in foster care due to the repeated severing of relationships. In the past few decades, however, I have also seen it in children who have had too many different caregivers, either from a day care with lots of turnover in new workers or in homes with too many changes in nannies. Babies thrive when they have a consistent loving relationship and can depend on their caregiver to be with them long-term.

The biggest problem with having a nanny is that it is expensive, especially for parents who have low paying jobs. In order to pay a nanny even the minimum wage for a full-time workweek, parents need to be making enough to cover all their expenses, plus have about $1500 per month left to pay the nanny. This is where some low interest parenting loans would come in handy.

One European model of an affordable way for children to be cared for in their homes is the au pair concept. An au pair is usually a college-aged student from another country who is given a private room, meals, and a small monetary allowance in exchange for caregiving the children and helping with some of the housework. The term "au pair" is French meaning "equal to," because the caregiver was intended to become a member of the family for the time she is living with them. The parents arrange their schedules so the au pair can have time to attend her own classes. She usually eats with the family and even joins in some of the family activities but spends time by herself in the evenings when the family has their own private time together.

In the past year, I created a similar situation in my own home to help care for my new puppy while I am working. I live near a large university and have rented two of my bedrooms to foreign students for many years after my own children left home. I currently have a student from Tibet who is here on a scholarship and needs a place to live for four years. I provide the room to her at a very discounted rate in exchange for her care of the puppy three afternoons per week. It has worked out wonderfully for all of us and the puppy is much happier than if she were left alone or in doggy day care. This seems like it could be a practical solution for many working parents who have an extra bedroom in their homes.

What is important to remember if your baby forms a close loving relationship with a nanny is that it will be extremely valuable to maintain that relationship for as long as possible. Even after the nanny is no longer working in your home, try to have her babysit for date nights, come to birthday or holiday celebrations, send postcards if she moves away, or in some way let your child know that when she loves someone they won't just disappear from her life.

## Single Mom Uses Live-in Family and Nanny

*Ann's story:*

*I was an RN in my mid-thirties when I shockingly discovered I was pregnant. Not being in a committed relationship with the man who fathered my child and finding out he was not interested in being a dad forced me to make the biggest decision of my life. Even though I had just been accepted into a sought-after nurse-midwifery master's degree program, I felt that at my age, if I ever wanted children, I could not turn this baby away and wait for a more convenient time. I embraced the pregnancy as an unexpected gift and became determined to find a way to adapt my life to meet this baby's needs.*

*During my pregnancy and after my little Ruby was born, I realized that as her sole parent it would be critical for us to have an especially close attachment to help her acquire the security she needed to build a strong inner foundation. I knew that this would only develop by spending as much time as possible with her whenever I could be there. From the beginning, I slept with Ruby in my bed and breastfed her whenever she desired throughout the night. I knew as a single working mom that I would have to return to my job when Ruby was only twelve weeks old, and that we would need lots of help from others. I just couldn't imagine leaving my tiny baby girl in a day care outside our home. So, I decided to cut down on expenses and bring other adults into our lives to help care for Ruby.*

*I moved out of my lovely townhouse, and my favorite age-mate cousin, Lisa, agreed to share the rent on a cheaper place. We moved in together when Ruby was six weeks old. It certainly was comforting to have someone else in the house. But Lisa had her own job, boyfriend, and busy life, and it became very clear that Ruby and I would need more help when I had to return to work. When Ruby was ten weeks old, my mom moved from her home a thousand miles away and came to live with us in our multigenerational home of related females. By sharing a house and childcare with both my cousin and mom, I was financially able to return to work part-time rather than full-time. Grandma Grace became Ruby's primary caregiver whenever I was working and would bring Ruby to me at least once a day to be nursed until she was eight months old. Besides it being the best food for Ruby, I knew that the breastfeeding bond was going to be an important part of our relationship. I was determined to keep up my milk supply and dutifully used a breast pump for eighteen months, pumping every three hours whenever we were apart.*

*Knowing that Grandma Grace had to return home after six months, when Ruby would be nine months old, I hired our nanny, Ana, one month before my mom needed to leave. Grandma cared for Ruby the first week while Ana watched and began to develop her own relationship with the baby. Ana took over the second week, and they alternated in this way for the month, which helped Ruby slowly transition from Grandma's care to Ana's care. At the end of Ruby's first year of life, I returned to school to finish my master's degree in nurse-midwifery, which I'd been able to defer for one year. As the sole bread earner, I still had to work while attending school, which meant I sometimes needed night and weekend care for Ruby. Ana made it possible by being wonderfully flexible. Ana had a husband and two daughters of her own, and they would often come to our house or Ruby would sometimes go to theirs. Our families comfortably became merged.*

*It was imperative to me that Ana be paid a living wage since she was helping raise my daughter, which I believe is the most important job in the world! Fifteen hundred dollars a month added significantly to the student loans I had to get, but I reminded myself that while I could pay back those loans over many decades, these early years of Ruby's life could never again be repeated. I knew how important it was to her development of trust, self-esteem, self-control, and the feeling of being loved.*

*I think my devotion to bed-sharing and breastfeeding has clearly paid off, since Ruby, now two and a half years old, still uses cuddling up and nursing as a comforting way to reconnect with me when I've been gone for an extended period of time. I know that these long absences are stressful for Ruby. She has always been much more needy and clingy the first day that I'm back home after a long shift. I've found that the best thing I can do is to just surrender and spend that entire first day doing whatever works to reconnect with her. I had to accept that during these years I would need to be devoted entirely to my career and my baby girl and would not have free time of my own to go out much or have a man in my life. Ruby requires as much of my unscheduled time as possible, and I've done my best to listen and try to meet her needs.*

*What has been most important to my success as a single parent from infancy through toddlerhood is having hands-on help from my extended family, flexible nanny care in my home, and a social support network of people both with and without kids. Other single moms also doing it solely on their own have been indispensible. It helps so much to commiserate about our unique challenges with others who totally understand.*

## Extended Family Support

*One family can influence another, then another, then ten,*
*One hundred, one thousand more, and the whole of society will benefit.*
—The Dalai Lama

One thing that all new families in the peaceful cultures of the world have in common is vast amounts of support from extended family and community. Raising a compassionate child is thought of as the responsibility of the village not just the parents. Gen Y parents and baby boomer grandparents are helping bring families in the US back together again. One consideration for a parent whose childcare costs are nearly half of her salary is that she could work only half-time with a grandparent or another extended family member covering the hours when she is at work, and she would still have the same amount of money at the end of the month.

When conducting the parent interviews I found it intriguing how three members of one extended family described their commitment to making great changes in order to be involved in their son and grandson's first few years of life. This family is doing a beautiful job of working together to ensure the baby is cared for at home by family members at all times, even though both parents need to be working full time. The following are interviews with the mom, dad, and one of the grandmothers, each telling the story from their own point of view. Recreating the extended family as caregivers along with much support from their closely bonded group of friends, who all have babies about the same age, is very similar to how humans throughout history have successfully met the needs of their young children.

## Extended Family Rallies to Help Working Couple

*Mama Ava's Story:*

*Dylan was born at the beginning of July and as a teacher I had the summer off. I wanted to stay home with my baby boy for as long as possible, so when the next school year began, I used the twelve weeks of paid sick leave that I had saved by never taking a day off during my previous six years of employment. I had been purposely saving that sick leave so I could have extra time off if I was lucky enough to ever have a baby. The paid leave took me to the end of November, but when it came time to return to work, I felt that neither Dylan nor I was ready to be apart. At that point I took four weeks of unpaid leave and we used money from our savings to cover expenses until the end of the year.*

*On January 3rd, when I returned to my classroom, it was the hardest day of my life. As I got in my car and drove away from home, my heart felt like a piece of it had been left behind. Even though I knew I would see Dylan at the end of the day, and that we were incredibly lucky to have both of Dylan's grandmothers willing to take care of him while my husband, Jonathan, and I were at work, it felt like part of my heart was being painfully* shattered. Jonathan's mother, Nana, had moved across the country in order to be Dylan's primary caregiver on Mondays, Tuesdays, and Wednesdays. My mother, Grammy, changed her work schedule; did her forty hour/week job in three ten-hour days and then would drive 120 miles to our home every Wednesday night, care for Dylan on Thursdays and Fridays, and drive back to her home on Saturday mornings, where my dad patiently waited for her. While this was a demanding schedule for Grammy, she cherished her time with Dylan and wouldn't have changed it for the world. I loved the fact that the grandmas came to our home so I didn't have to pack things up early every morning and take Dylan anywhere. He would still be in his jammies when his Nana arrived or Grammy emerged from our guest room and breast milk for the day was conveniently waiting in the refrigerator. Dylan was able to stay in his own home surrounded by the toys, bed, and pets with which he was so familiar and happy.

The only way I was emotionally able to walk out the door every morning and go to work was knowing that Dylan was being cared for by someone who truly loved him deeply and put her entire heart into making sure that all of his physical, emotional, and developmental needs were being met every moment of the day. It meant the world to me knowing that when Dylan was held, he was feeling love from one of his grandmas and when he was being fed, rocked to sleep, held quietly reading books, going out on adventures, or whatever the day brought, it always was filled with love. I also felt such a sense of relief knowing that the grandmas would adjust their days based on Dylan's needs. For example, if he'd had an especially sleepless night, rough time with teething, or was a touch under the weather, they would always give him the extra comfort he needed. Each day I had the grandmas write down information about their time spent with Dylan. They documented his basic needs, like when and how much he ate and slept, how he was feeling, what he enjoyed, his first milestones, and what activities they did throughout the day. When I returned home from work, after tons of huge hugs and kisses with my baby boy, one of my favorite things was sitting down with either Nana or Grammy and hearing about their day in detail, including looking at all the photos and videos taken that day of Dylan. These debriefing times really helped me feel like I wasn't missing out on too much, although sometimes I still felt sad that I wasn't the one getting to have those experiences with my son.

*If we had paid parental leave in this country, I would definitely have delighted in spending Dylan's infancy and toddlerhood with him. I think these times are so important in terms of creating a foundation for who a person becomes. Jonathan and I are wanting to have another baby in the next few years and really worry about how I will be able to stay home even as long as I did with Dylan since I won't be able to save up six more years of sick leave. We've been thinking of starting a maternity leave savings account with an automatic monthly transfer in order to build some financial reserve so our future baby can have me at home for as long as possible. With only twelve weeks of unpaid leave, there is no way at the current time that I'll be able to stay home very long with our next baby.*

*Jonathan has been such an incredibly supportive husband and father with hands-on care of Dylan from the beginning. I especially appreciate that in the evenings after he gets home from work, he understands that I really need special time to reconnect with Dylan. On most nights Jonathan will take the lead in preparing dinner and does the majority of dinner cleanup, as well, so that I can just be with the baby. No matter how exhausted I am from the stresses of working and not getting much sleep, those evenings are so important for me to spend with the baby. Although Jonathan has been very involved in every aspect of Dylan's direct caregiving, including taking turns during middle of the night and early morning wake ups, Dylan still often wants to be with me. I think it is hard at times for Jonathan to see the special bond that a mother and baby have, but he does understand completely how important it is for a baby to feel closely connected to his mommy. Jonathan still makes a point of having special quality time with Dylan. They frequently read books, play the piano and sing together in the basement, and Jonathan is always telling Dylan, "Daddy loves you!" Watching my husband turn into an amazing father is one of the most beautiful things I have ever experienced.*

*Even though having a baby has taken away from the time Jonathan and I used to have individually and as a couple, and I don't have as much nurturing energy left for my husband, I actually feel like it has brought us much closer than we were before. It has turned us into a team working together for the common goal of a healthy child and happy family. I feel really lucky to have such an amazing support system. My husband, mom, mother-in-*

law, extended family, and incredibly supportive moms group with babies the same age as Dylan have been essential to my feelings of competence, composure, and success as a working mom.

*Daddy Jonathan's Story:*

Although I have been involved in hands-on caregiving of my son, Dylan, since the moment of his birth, the thing that feels most important in terms of staying really connected with him is our one-on-one play times. On the weekends, his mom, Ava, and I alternate who gets up early in the morning with Dylan and lets the other one sleep in. Even though it's so hard to get out of bed, I find those hours between wake-up and Dylan's first nap of the day to be really special. Just hanging out, playing together, encouraging him to crawl, walk, or throw a ball is really fun. Our favorite thing is going down to my music room in the basement. He loves to sit on my lap and play the piano or guitar—today we played Beatles tunes all morning. Dylan really enjoys listening to music and being around people when they are making music.

When Dylan was born, I tried to take two weeks off, but I work at a very small company and my boss said he could only spare for me not to be working for one week. He did let me work from home during the second week and gave me a fully-paid leave. I'm fortunate to have a boss who is genuinely supportive of dads being involved in their kids' lives and is super good about offering flexibility in terms of hours and days worked. It definitely makes me feel more loyal to him, because he's so accommodating to my family. I am very clear that my child is first and then my career.

My mom was a stay-at-home mom until I was in middle school and I felt really lucky to have her at home for so long. I can't imagine sending Dylan to day care, it seems like it would be really scary for a little kid. Ultimately day care is a business doing it for money, which is so much different from grandmothers who are doing it for love. It is very fortunate that my mom was financially able and willing to move across the country, get an apartment in town, and take care of Dylan three days a week last winter and spring when Ava had to return to work. Now, my dad is getting ready to retire, and is trying to sell the family home back east so he and my mom can move out here permanently and share in our lives. I'm also extremely *thankful that Ava's mom has been willing to arrange her work schedule and drive over a hundred miles to our home in order to take care of Dylan two days a week.*

*I think it is really important for babies to feel closely bonded to their moms. From the beginning I have tried to help out whenever I could around the house so Ava could have as much time as possible with the Dylan. After Ava went back to work, I usually cooked and cleaned the kitchen every night. It's the little things like cleaning, doing the dishes, and keeping things easy around the house that can make a big difference. I have felt zero competition with Ava about the fact that as a baby Dylan usually prefers to be with her. Whenever he wants to be nursed I always take him to right to his mom, especially during the night, rather than trying to give him a bottle of breast milk. I totally get it when Dylan cries and wants his mommy, I mean lots of times I want my mommy, too! I know when he grows older he'll get to a stage when he'll want to spend lots more time with me. I have a very diverse skill set that will be interesting to him and help him bond more with me in a different sort of way. I'm really looking forward to playing music together and already have gotten a lot of science experiments lined up that I can't wait to show him.*

*Right now I am feeling really good about being able to financially provide for my family. It may be a pretty traditional father-type role, but it is one that feels important. I'm lucky to have a pretty well-paying job and it is nice that we're quite comfortable and don't have to worry about finances. That way we can focus on Dylan and what makes him happy and if he needs new clothes or something, we can get them with very little stress about it. This is a big part of feeling relaxed as a family, because financial worries can really cause a lot of stress. I don't actually know how other dads feel about all of these issues because guys don't usually talk about these things. I mean, when Ava gets together with other moms they talk about everything, but as dads, we just sorta hang out and swap stories.*

*The biggest change in my relationship with Ava is that we used to have a lot of good times going out together to fun little spots in town, but now we've become more homebodies. Babies can't really be taken out at night, and we want to be with him, so we've probably only gone out on maybe three dates since he was born thirteen months ago. It's really changed how we spend time from doing couple things to being a family. But that's the name of the game right now.*

*The absolute toughest part of parenting for me has been the lack of sleep. I'm someone who loves to sleep and used to get ten hours a night, and have had to cut back to maybe seven or eight on really good nights. Dylan's finally getting a bit better now at sleeping, but for that first year it was pretty rough. Even though people tell you about it and you see it coming, there is truly no way to understand until you actually experience it. I was exhausted all the time, and it was sometimes difficult to even stay focused at work when I was so tired. But I know it's definitely all about the long game and that I will get to sleep-in at some point again in my life.*

*The truly best part of being a dad is Dylan. When I look at my son, he's so cute and awesome. I've never really been around very young children before, but Dylan is so incredible. We're really stoked; he's such a wonderful little kid! I'm certainly looking forward to watching him keep growing. I sincerely believe that when kids get their early needs met, it can make the whole world a better place.*

*From Grammy's Point of View:*

*The two and a half weeks that began with supporting my daughter, Ava, in her attempted home birth, unbelievably difficult labor, transfer to the hospital, unexpected emergency cesarean, then living in their home, help- ing care for them as they bonded as a new family, and my own intense attachment to my first grandchild, Dylan, has changed me forever. I love being a grandmother!*

*It has been a joy watching Ava and Dylan's dad, Jonathan, as parents; the way they are with Dylan is truly exceptional. From the moment Dylan was born after a traumatically difficult emergency cesarean birth, Jonathan ripped open the front of his hospital gown and held the newborn reassur- ingly against his bare chest for the first forty minutes, while doctors worked to help Ava recover. As soon as Dylan was placed at his mommy's breast the fear from the frightening birth was transformed, Ava's eyes began glowing and I saw Dylan look up and smile at his mommy when he was less than an hour old. We all knew at that moment that Dylan was actually "born at home," because his home is in his parents arms and hearts. That birth expe- rience, which had been so different than they had planned, assured me that they were truly ready to be parents, able to set expectations aside and make the most of whatever happened in their child's life.*

*Ava was as prepared for mothering as any woman could possibly be, but she couldn't even imagine how powerful her attachment to Dylan would feel. One of the first things she said to me about that bond was, "Now I understand how you feel, Mom. How will I ever let him go?" From the beginning, Jonathan was a hands-on, do everything but feed the baby kind of dad. There were even some things like swaddling or bouncing on the yoga ball, like Mom had done while pregnant, that Dad mastered to comfort Dylan. As an infant, the parents were deeply committed to skin-to-skin contact, constantly holding Dylan, bed sharing, listening, and responding to his every cue. I don't think he was ever out of someone's arms during the early weeks of his life. As a result of their attentive behavior, I have never actually heard Dylan cry.*

*Dylan is a gentle, loving soul. Spending time with him is simply delightful. It's hard to tell exactly how much is due to the incredibly skilled and loving parenting he receives, and how much is due to his innate personality, but he is now a most amazing thirteen-month-old. Dylan has always had someone trying to understand and respond to his needs. When he wants something, it is very easy to read his cues because he's so present and responsive. The way Dylan reaches out and connects with others physically and emotionally opens hearts and engages cooperation.*

*One of my most cherished memories is of holding Dylan as a newborn while he was falling asleep and feeling his tiny hand gently touching my chest. His energy was so very tender and peaceful. At that moment I could feel the beginning of a very deep lifelong bond. This early attachment to Dylan made me realize that I wanted to be involved in his everyday life and become a primary caregiver when Ava had to return to work after six months of maternity leave. I talked with my employer and developed an alternative work plan. They let me change to three ten-hour days per week, working Monday through Wednesday. This allowed me leave on Wednesday evenings, drive the 120 miles to Ava and Jonathan's home, care for Dylan on Thursdays and Fridays, and return back home on Saturdays. Although, as a grandmother this has been an extraordinary experience, the employment and commuting piece have been extremely difficult. Making the transition to thirty hours a week while still trying to get the same forty-hour workload* done, and driving in the middle of winter on dark, rainy, snowy, and icy roads was grueling.

Ava and Jonathan's welcoming ritual of always having the family sitting at the dinner table waiting for me with a hot meal helped all my stress from work and the drive instantly fall away. Once I was there it was truly wonderful! After dinner, the three of them would go off and have their evening time together while I settled into being in their home. Ava was transitioning from a full-time stay-at-home mom to being a full-time working-mom; this was very hard for her because she missed Dylan terribly while she was away. It became a priority for all of us to make sure that Ava could be with Dylan one hundred percent of the time after she got home from work. I would do as much as I could to help make life easier for them, like doing the laundry, cleaning, shopping, and preparing meals, so they could have more time with Dylan and each other. In the evenings, I tried to be as unobtrusive as possible so they could have time and space to reconnect with each other after being apart all day.

It has been wonderful witnessing the kind of parents "the kids" have become. I have loved seeing that Jonathan is such an involved Dad. He was always on "first call" at night. Dylan, six months old at that time, was starting out each night in his own room, but when he stirred during the night, as observed on the video monitor next to the bed, Jonathan would go to comfort him. If Dylan wanted to be nursed, Jonathan took Dylan back to bed and into Ava's arms. It is such a comfort to know how Jonathan and Ava delight in parenting and how they talk to each other, with so much joy, respect, and love for Dylan. I believe that if we were all treated this way from the beginning of life, it would truly be a very different world.

Dylan, as yet, has never been cared for by anyone other than a family member.

On Mondays, Tuesdays, and Wednesdays, Jonathan's mom takes care of Dylan. Ava created a logbook that explains their parenting beliefs and practices along with a daily log that we grandmas fill out about all of the things Dylan and we did during the day. I love to take lots of videos each day of the many adventures he and I do together to share with them in the evenings. In order to help with continuity of care, the four of us on his caregiving team go out to dinner once a month to talk about Dylan and our experiences of *caring for him. As grandmothers, being involved in primary caregiving is such a great opportunity to see our own adult son or daughter in a new way, and it's creating a new closer relationship with each of them. Being elders we have confidence that most things will work out with our grandson and are freed from so much of the anxiety that we felt as young moms. For example, I don't worry if Dylan doesn't take a long nap, have enough tummy time, or gets a rash that it will have long-term consequences. This allows me to just enjoy every precious moment with him.*

*Being a primary caregiver has been such a wonderful experience for me that I am looking forward to doing it again next year once Ava returns to teaching in September. I had been financially preparing to retire in a couple of years, but since my employer is no longer willing to offer me the same thirty-hour workweek, I've decided to retire two years earlier than expected. No longer having the work pressures and such an exhausting schedule will be a great relief. I am aware of how fortunate I am to be participating daily in my daughter's family and couldn't be happier. I'm in awe of how sharing the experience of us both being mothers has deepened and transformed my relationship with Ava. I have so much respect for the woman she has become, choices she has made, and loving family she is creating.*

*As a grandmother, my greatest challenge is not to question my daughter when she is parenting differently than I did. When Ava wants something done with Dylan, even when I don't understand it, I do it her way. We do have a "one time only" rule in our family that if one of us has a strong opinion about something—that person gets to clearly express it once, have others listen without any argument, and then just leave it alone. Sometimes after consideration it is brought back up by the listener and discussed, and other times it is never mentioned again, but the initiator experiences a sense of relief that at least there was a chance to be heard. "One time only" has served our family well over the years.*

*Dylan has brought our whole extended family closer, from the celebration of his birth that began with all of us together in that hospital room, to a new openness that I feel with my daughter and see between Ava and her siblings, who all adore Dylan. Since I am gone from my husband three days a week, we have developed some rituals to keep us connected. Every morning after Ava and Jonathan leave for work, I take a video of Dylan and send it to his Grandpa. Grandpa is very loving and sweet with Dylan, and seems softer and more relaxed than he was with our own kids when they were babies. I had thought my husband would join me in helping care for Dylan at least a few times a month, but Grandpa's involved in his own work and telecommutes from home. When I return on Saturday mornings, he is very eager to see me, and delights in hearing stories and seeing videos of how things are going with our kids and grandson. He's very proud of what I am doing, and even though we spend less time together, it seems to have created a special positive energy between us, and a new kind of intimacy. We love sharing in our children's lives; watching them become parents has been unbelievably wonderful.*

## Mindful Parenting Grows Kind Kids

*In order to change the world...*
*Most important is maximum affection and time with your children.*
—The Dalai Lama

Peaceful cultures have shown and early brain research has confirmed that it is indeed possible to grow people with more abilities to calm their intense emotions, use better judgment, creatively problem solve, and have increased capacities to be compassionate, empathetic, generous, and loving. In my forty years of observing parents throughout the world, it became clear that the attentive, responsive nurturing of infants and toddlers in peaceful societies is significantly different from that in other cultures. Great emphasis is placed on positive birthing experiences and honoring rituals to ensure that infants are welcomed with much gentleness and cherishing. Practices that promote attachment and trust begin at the moment of birth and are continued throughout the first few years of life during the greatest period of brain growth. Closely attached toddlers want to please their primary caregivers and as their consciences develop they are helped to listen inside when making decisions of right or wrong. Secure, competent, joyful, and kind children are the result of such parenting.

The Mindful Parenting practices for infants and toddlers presented in this book can help parents replicate the compassionate treatment of young children that is observed in peaceful cultures. The complexity of parenting each very different child along with the infinite number of stresses in our fast-paced lifestyles makes it absolutely impossible to parent without many doubts and regrets. But you will successfully raise a delightful child if you remember two of the most important parenting practices from all those that have been discussed. (1) Always listen and respond to what your baby is trying to tell you; she will truly be your finest teacher of how she needs to be parented, and (2) When your relationship with your child becomes disconnected, do your very best to emotionally reconnect with her as soon as you can. Please also remember to be kind to yourself and take those time-outs when *you* need them. Don't burden yourself so much that you aren't the caring parent you want to be, and forgive yourself for acting in ways that you swore you never would. When you apologize to your child it teaches them how to better accept their own mistakes and how to admit when they need to "push the refresh button."

Many modern parents are making meaningful changes in their life priorities in order to better meet the early needs of their infants and toddlers. If all babies had the kind of start in life where they felt nurtured and cherished by mindful parents who were attentive, responsive, kind, and loving, what a different world this could be! This next generation of children could have better skills at negotiating and compromising, which would be especially valuable in working cooperatively with the interwoven global community on environmental, economic, and peacekeeping solutions. A world beyond war will require people who are more empathetic, trusting, and creative at finding solutions that benefit the greater good of humanity and our earth. There are so many different cultures, beliefs, and ways of life, but all humans want basically the same things for themselves and their children. We all desire to have freedom, safety, basic needs met, connection to a trusted group of family and friends, to be heard, respected, appreciated, cared for, and loved. Growing kind kids who have the mental and emotional ability to build bridges between those with ideological differences could truly help this generation become the peacemakers we need to support the survival of our species and this beautiful planet we call home.

*You are a beloved of the universe.*
*You are as beautiful as the sunrise, and as ancient as the stars.*
*You are a spark of divine love in human form.*
*Through you goodness and light flow into this world.*
—Laurel Bleadon-Maffei

# APPENDIX

# Indicators of Children in Crisis

How do we know that current parenting practices in the US are not meeting the needs of our children? Unfortunately, we do not have to look far to find sobering statistics that clearly portray the seriousness of the mental health crisis American children are presently experiencing from the beginning of conception. In the United States:

- Twenty-eight percent of new mothers are subject to physical violence while pregnant.[1]
- The number of premature babies born has increased by thirty-six percent since the 1980s. More than half a million premature babies are born every year.[2]
- Although ranking in the top thirty-one high-income industrialized countries, there are forty-five countries in the world that have a lower infant mortality rate than does the US.[3]
- There are one million cases of serious child abuse and neglect reported each year.[4]
- Half a million preschool children must at times take care of themselves.[5]
- Twenty percent of school-aged kids between six and twelve years old reported not having had even a ten-minute conversation with either parent in the previous month.[6]
- One in every five children is diagnosed with a psychiatric or psychological problem.[7]
- In the past five years, emergency rooms have been swamped with a sixty percent increase of parents bringing in children suffering from depression, anxiety, and suicide attempts.[8]
- Children are receiving an increasing number of diagnoses and medication for: depression, obsessive-compulsive disorder, anxiety disorders, conduct disorders, anorexia nervosa, sleep disorders, and phobias.[9]

- Ninety percent of all the medications in the world that are given to children for mental health issues are used in this country.[10]
- Children have less respect for authority; they are harder to teach and manage at home and in schools. There is increased bullying, with children even murdering other children.[11]
- Thirteen million children will be bullied in the US this year.[12]
- Mass shootings of children killing adults and other children has significantly increased over the past fifteen years.
- Suicide of children from ages five to fifteen has doubled in the past twenty years, and tripled in the past fifty years.[13]
- Suicide is the third leading cause of death among teenagers and the second leading cause of death among college-aged youth.[14]
- Homicide is the fourth leading cause of death in children under age four, and is the second leading cause of death for kids between the ages of fifteen and twenty-four years.[15]
- There are approximately twelve gun deaths *daily* of people under the age of nineteen.[16]
- The overall firearm-related death rate among children under age fifteen is nearly *twelve times higher* than among children in *all the other twenty-five industrialized countries combined.*[17]

William Damon, a leading scholar of human development, points out that, "Practically all of the indicators of youth health and behavior have declined year by year for well over a generation. None have improved. The litany is now so well known, that it is losing its power to shock."[18]

It is imperative, however, that we continue to be shocked by such statistics! Most Americans have been unaware of how bad things have become for our kids and are at a loss as to how we can begin repairing the damage. However, the children in our country need us to listen to their pain, and not disregard this frightening and heartbreaking trend.

# Notes

## Introduction

1. Piero Ferrucci, *The Power of Kindness: The Unexpected Benefits of Leading a Compassionate Life* (London, England: Penguin Books, 2006).

## Chapter 1

1. Erik Erikson, *Childhood and Society* (New York City: NY: WW Norton & Company, 1950).
2. Robert Knox Dentan, *The Semai: A Nonviolent People of Malaya* (New York: Holt, Rinehart and Winston,1968).
3. Riane Eisler, *The Chalice and the Blade* (New York City. NY: HarperCollins, 1988).
4. *Women of Tibet: Gyalyum Chemo The Great Mother*, directed by Rosemary Rawcliff (San Francisco, CA: Frame of Mind Films, 2006), DVD.
5. Ann Hubbell Maiden and Edie Farwell, *The Tibetan Art of Parenting: From Before Conception Through Early Childhood* (Somerville, MA: Wisdom Publications, 1997), 99.
6. *Kundun,* Directed by Martin Scorsese (Burbank, CA: Touchstone Pictures. 1997). DVD.
7. *Women of Tibet*, Rawcliff.
8. *Kundun,* Scorsese.
9. Maiden and Farwell, *The Tibetan Art of Parenting.*
10. Bruce H. Lipton, PhD, *The Biology of Belief: Unleashing the Power of Consciousness, Matter & Miracle* (Santa Rosa, CA: Mountain of Love/Elite Books, 2005).
11. Maiden and Farwell, *The Tibetan Art of Parenting*, 43.
12. Maiden and Farwell, *The Tibetan Art of Parenting.*

13. Maiden and Farwell, *The Tibetan Art of Parenting*, 113.
14. Maiden and Farwell, *The Tibetan Art of Parenting*, 131.
15. Oliver Follmi and Danielle Follmi, *Offerings: Spiritual Wisdom to Change Your Life* (New York City, NY: Stewart, Tabori & Chang, 2002).
16. Rinchen Khando Choegyal, personal interview (Dharmsala, India, December 1994).
17. Maiden and Farwell, *The Tibetan Art of Parenting*, ix.
18. Choegyal, personal interview.
19 Wikipedia, "Gross National Happiness," last Modified August 10, 2015, http: //en.wikipedia.org/wiki/Gross_national_happiness.
20. Russ Carpenter and Blyth Carpenter, *The Blessings of Bhutan* (Honolulu, HI: University of Hawai'i Press, 2002), 155–157.
21. Mimi Lhamu, MD, personal interview (Thimphu, Bhutan, February 25, 2004).
22. Charlotte Peterson, PhD, personal observations (Bali, Indonesia, 2002).
23. Wayan Ratna, personal interview (Ubud, Bali, Indonesia, August, 2002).
24. Ketut Karta, personal interview (Penestanan, Bali, Indonesia, August 2002).
25. Nyoman Gandri, personal interview (Payogan, Bali, Indonesia, July 2002).
26. Gandri, personal interview.
27. Made Narok, personal interview (Penestanan, Bali, Indonesia, July 2002).
28. Norihiro Kato, "Japan's Break with Peace," *The New York Times*, July 16, 2014.
29. Naho Kikuchi, personal interview (Tokyo, Japan, September 2002).
30. Kikuchi, personal interview.

## Chapter 2

1. Meredith F. Small, *Kids: How Biology and Culture Shape the Way We Raise Young Children* (New York City, NY: Anchor Books, 2001), 3.

2. Sarah Blaffer Hrdy, *Mother Nature: Maternal Instincts and How They Shape The Human Species* (New York City, NY: Ballantine Publishing Group, 2000),161.

3. Blaffer Hrdy, *Mother Nature*, 162.

4. S. P. Mendoza and W.A. Mason, "Attachment Relationships in New World Primates," in *The Integrative Neurobiology of Affiliation*, ed. C. S. Carter, I .I. Lederhendler, and B. Kirkpatrick (Cambridge, MA: MIT Press, 1999), 93–100.

5. Susan Allport, *A Natural History of Parenting: A Naturalist Looks at Parenting In the Animal World and Ours* (Bloomington, IN: iUniverse, 2003),165–173.

6. Barbara Wootton, Mary D. Salter Ainsworth, R. G. Andry, Robert G. Harlow, S. Lebovici, Margaret Mead, and Diane G. Prugh, "Deprivation of Maternal Care: A Reassessment of Its Effects," (Geneva, Switzerland: *World Health Organization, Public Health Papers*, No.14 1962), 255-266. http://apps.who.int/iris/handle/10665/37819.

7. Allport, *A Natural History of Parenting*, 168.

8. Inge Bretherton, "The Origins of Attachment Theory: John Bowlby and Mary Ainsworth," *Developmental Psychology 28* (1992): 759–775.

9. Susan Allport, *A Natural History of Parenting*, 179.

10. Small, *Kids*, 47.

11. Joseph Chilton Pearce and Bruce H. Lipton, "The Evolution of Biology and Development of Spiritual Intelligence" (APPPAH Post Congress Workshop, San Francisco, CA, December 10, 2001).

12. Marshall H. Klaus, MD and Phyllis H. Klaus, *Your Amazing Newborn* (New York City, NY: HarperCollins Publishers, 1998), 24.

13. Marshall H. Klaus, MD and John H. Kennel, *Maternal-infant Bonding* (St. Louis, MO: C.V. Mosby Co., 1976).

14. *Delivery Self-Attachment.* directed by Lennart Righard (Los Angeles, CA: Geddes Productions. 1995), Video.

15. Baby Friendly USA, "Implementing the UNICEF/WHO Baby Friendly Hospital Initiative in the U.S.," last modified 2012, http://www.babyfriendlyusa.org.

16. Blaffer Hrdy *Mother Nature,*,130–131.

17. Patrick M. Houser, "The Science of Father Love," Association for Prenatal and Perinatal Psychology and Health, 2011. https://birthpsychology.com/free-article/science-father-love.
18. Patrick M. Houser, "Breast is Best . . . for Dads too!" La Leche League Magazine: *New Beginnings*, August 2009.
19. Jack Heinowitz, *Fathering Right from the Start: Straight Talk about Pregnancy, Birth and Beyond* (Novato, CA: New World Library, 2001).
20. Houser, "Breast is Best."
21. Houser, "The Science of Father Love."
22. Blaffer Hrdy *Mother Nature*.
23. Kikuchi, personal interview.
24. Samuel J. Formon, "Infant Feeding in the 20th Century: Formula and Beikost." *Journal of Nutrition* 131 (2001): 4095–4205.
25. Blaffer Hrdy *Mother Nature*, 11.
26. Robert Karen, *Becoming Attached: First Relationships and How They Shape Our Capacity to Love* (New York City, NY: Oxford University Press, 1994).
27. Sobonfu E. Somé, *Welcoming Spirit Home: Ancient African Teachings to Celebrate Children and Community* (Novato, CA: New World Library, 1999).
28. Houser, "The Science of Father Love."
29. S. E. Taylor et al., "Female Responses to Stress: Tend and Befriend, Not Fight or Flight," *Psychological Review* 107, no. 3 (2000): 411–429.
30. Taylor et al., "Female Responses to Stress."
31. Mary E. Clark, *In Search of Human Nature* (New York City, NY: Routledge, 2002).

## Chapter 3

1. Jack Newman, MD, "The Importance of Skin to Skin Contact," International Breast-feeding Center, 2009. http://www.nbci.ca/index.php?option=com_content&id=82: the-importance-of-skin-to-skin-contact-&Itemid=17.
2. Houser, "The Science of Father Love."

3. Association for Prenatal and Perinatal Psychology and Health, "Welcome Your Baby In With 60 Minutes, Skin-to-Skin," (Advocate Reference Card, 2010). http://www.birthpsychology.com.
4. Infant Massage USA, "Benefits of Infant Massage," 2011. www.infant-massageusa /learn-to-massage-your-baby/benefits-of-infantmassage/.
5. A. M. Widstrom, W. Wahlburg and A.S. Matthiesen, "Short-term effects of early suckling and touch of the nipple on maternal behavior," *Early Human Development* 21 (1990): 153–163.
6. Ratna, personal interview.
7. Gandri, personal interview.
8. Lhamu, personal interview
9. Formon, "Infant Feeding in the 20th Century.
10. Desiree Nelson, RN, IBCLC, written personal communication, December 12, 2011.
11. L. M. Gartner et al., Policy Statement: "Breastfeeding and the use of human milk," *Pediatrics* 115 no.2 (2005): 496–506.
12. World Health Organization, "Nutrition: Exclusive Breast-feeding," 2011. http://www.who.int/nutrition/topics/exclusive_breast-feeding/en/.
13. World Health Organization, "Global Strategy for Infant and Young Child Feeding," (Geneva, Switzerland: World Health Organization and UNICEF, 2003).
14. Robin Lim, personal interview (Banjar Nyuh Kuning, Bali, March 31, 2004).
15. M. M. Vennemann et. al., "Does Breast-feeding Reduce the Risk of Sudden Infant Death Syndrome," *Pediatrics,* 123 (2009): e406–e410.
16. American Academy of Pediatrics, Resolution #67SC, "Divesting From Formula Marketing in Pediatric Care," Breastfeeding Initiatives, November 25, 2011. https: //www2.aap.org/breastfeeding/files/pdf/DivestingfromFormulaMarketinginPediatricCare.pdf.
17. World Health Organization, "Nutrition."
18. Baby Friendly USA, "Implementing the UNICEF/WHO Baby Friendly Hospital Initiative in the U.S."
19. Agency for Healthcare Research and Quality, "Breastfeeding and Maternal and Infant Health Outcomes in Developed Countries," evidence report April 2007. http//www.ahrq.gov/clinic.epcarch.htm.

20. Agency for Healthcare Research and Quality, "Breastfeeding and Maternal and Infant Health Outcomes in Developed Countries."

21. H. S. Littman, VanderBrug Medendorp, and J. Goldfarb. "The Decision to Breastfeed: The Importance of Fathers' Approval." *Clinical Pediatrics, 33, no.*4 (1994): 214–219.

22. Oliver Follmi and Danielle Follmi. *Offerings: Spiritual Wisdom to Change Your Life* (New York City, NY: Stewart, Tabori & Chang, 2002).

23. Kikuchi, personal interview.

24. Gandri, personal interview.

25. Lhamu, personal interview

26. G. Morelli et al., "Cultural variation in infants' sleeping arrangements: Questions of independence," *Developmental Psychology* 28 (1992): 604–613.

27. James J. McKenna, PhD, *Sleeping with Your Baby: A Parent's Guide to Cosleeping* (Washington, DC: Platypus Media; 1 edition, 2007), 58.

28. McKenna, *Sleeping with Your Baby,* 32.

29. McKenna, *Sleeping with Your Baby,* 33.

30. James J. McKenna et al., "Sleep and Arousal Patterns of Co-Sleeping Human Mother-Infant Pairs: A Preliminary Physiological Study with Implications for the Study of the Sudden Infant Death Syndrome (SIDS)," *American Journal of Physical Anthropology,* 82 no.3 (1990): 331-347.

31. McKenna, *Sleeping with Your Baby,* 37.

32. McKenna, *Sleeping with Your Baby,* 21.

33. James J. McKenna, PhD and Lee T. Gettler, "Mother-Infant Cosleeping with Breastfeeding in the Western Industrialized Context: A Bicultural Perspective," in *Textbook of Human Lactation,* eds. T. W. Hale and P. E. Hartmann, (Amarillo, TX: Hale Publishing, 2007).

34. McKenna, *Sleeping with Your Baby,* 22.

35. McKenna, *Sleeping with Your Baby,* 61–70.

36. Healthy Babies, Healthy Communities, "Safe Sleep." Flyer by a grant from the CJ Foundation for SIDS, (Lane County, Oregon, 2009). www.lanecounty.org /prevention.

37. McKenna, *Sleeping with Your Baby,* 61–70.

38. Healthy Babies, Healthy Communities, "Safe Sleep."

39. McKenna, *Sleeping with Your Baby,* p. 77.
40. Rob Reiner, *The First Years Last Forever* (2005).
41. M. Crawford, "Parenting Practices in the Basque Country: Implications of Infant and Childhood Sleeping Location for Personality Development." *Ethos* 22, no. 1 (1994): 42–82.
42. The First Years Last Forever 2005.
43. Lhamu, personal interview.
44. McKenna, *Sleeping with Your Baby,* p. 77.
45. The First Years Last Forever 2005.
46. Erickson, *Childhood and Society.*
47. Emmett L. Holt, MD, *The Care and Feeding of Children: A Catechism for the Use of Mothers and Children's Nurse,* Public domain in the USA, (1907).
48. William Sears, MD, Robert Sears, MD, James Sears, MD, and Martha Sears, RN. *The Baby Sleep Book: The Complete Guide to a Good Night's Rest for the Whole Family,* (Boston, MA: Little, Brown and Company, 2005).
49. Australian Association of Infant Mental Health, Position Paper 1: "Controlled Crying," March 2004. http://www.aaimhi.org/inewsfiles/controlled_crying.pdf.
50. McKenna, *Sleeping with Your Baby,* 38.
51. Klaus and Klaus, *Your Amazing Newborn,* 24–37.
52. Karta, personal interview.
53. Narok, personal interview.
54. K. Lee, "The Crying Patterns of Korean infants & related factors," *Developmental Medicine & Child Neurology* 36 (1994): 601–607.
55. *Reducing Infant Mortality,* directed by Debby Takikawa, (Santa Barbara, CA: Hana Peace Works, 2009), DVD.
56. National Institute of Child Health and Human Development 2013.
57. Guttmacher Institute, "Facts on Unintended Pregnancy in the United States," January 2012. www.guttmacher.org/pubs/FB-Unintended-Pregnancy-US.html.
58. National Institute of Child Health and Human Development, "High C-section rate may have something to do with impatience," *Los Angeles Times,* August 30, 2010.

59. Nathanael Johnson, "As early elective births increase so do health risks for mother, child," California Watch: December 26, 2010. http://californiawatch.org.

60. Pat MacEnulty, "Oh Baby: Ina May Gaskin on the Medicalization of Birth," *The Sun,* January 2012, 5–13.

61. Lim, personal interview.

62. International Childbirth Education Association, *Cesarean Fact Sheet,* 1995-1998. http://www.childbirth.org/section/CSFact.html.

63. Klaus and Kennel, *Maternal-infant Bonding.*

64. Johnson, "As early elective births increase so do health risks for mother, child."

65. Sarah J. Buckley, MD, *Gentle Birth, Gentle Mothering: The Wisdom and Science of Gentle Choices in Pregnancy, Birth, and Parenting* (Australia: One Moon Press, 2005).

66. Buckley, *Gentle Birth, Gentle Mothering.*

67. Daniel Siegel, MD and Mary Hartzell, Med, *Parenting From The Inside Out* (New York City, NY: Penguin Group (USA) Inc., 2003).

68. Jeane Rhodes, PhD and Michael J. Kloepfer, *The Birth of Hope: a unique novel* (Charleston, SC: CreateSpace Independent Publishing Platform, 2009).

69. Wendy Davis, PhD, "Perinatal Mood Disorders," (Presentation, Lane County, Oregon: May 8, 2006). http://www.babybluesconnection.org.

70. Davis, "Perinatal Mood Disorders."

## Chapter 4

1. Lawrence Balter, *Parenthood in America: An Encyclopedia, Volume 1* (Santa Barbara, CA: ABC-CLIO, Inc., 2000).

2. Brené Brown, PhD, *The Gifts of Imperfection: Let Go of Who You Think You're Supposed to Be and Embrace Who You Are* (Center City, MN: Hazelden, 2010).

3. Eric Page, "Benjamin Spock, World's Pediatrician, Dies at 94," *The New York Times,* Learning Network, March 17, 1998. http://learning. blogs.nytimes.com/.

4. Mary E. Clark, personal conversation. Eugene, OR, 2011.

5. Michael Pearls, and Debi Pearls, *To Train Up A Child* (Pleasantville, TN: No Greater Joy Ministries, 1994).
6. Lynn Harris, "Spare the quarter-inch plumbing supply line, spoil the child," May 25, 2006. http://www.salon.com/life/feature/2006/05/25/the_pearls
7. Gary Ezzo, *On Becoming Babywise* (Sisters, Oregon: Multnomah Publishers, 1998).
8. Gary Ezzo and Robert Bucknam, *On Becoming Babywise: Giving Your Infant the Gift of Nighttime Sleep* (Sisters, Oregon: Multnomah Publishers, 2006).
9. Matthew Aney, MD, "Babywise advice linked to dehydration, failure to thrive," 1995. http://www.ezzo.info/resources/timeline/81-timeline/107-babywise-advice-linked-to-dehydration-failure-to-thrive.
10. Steve Rein, "Evaluating Ezzo Programs," last modified 2013. http://www.ezzo.info.
11. American Academy of Pediatrics, Policy Statement: "Breastfeeding and the Use of Human Milk," *Pediatrics* 115 no. 2 (February 2005): 496–506.
12. Balter, *Parenthood in America*, 178.
13. Benjamin Spock, *The Common Sense Book of Baby and Child Care* (New York City, NY: Duell, Sloan, and Pearce, 1946).
14. Silvia M. Bell and Mary D. Salter Ainsworth, "Infant crying and maternal responsiveness," *Child Development* 43 (1972): 1171–90.
15. K. Lee, "The Crying Patterns of Korean Infants & Related Factors," *Developmental Medicine & Child Neurology* 36 (1994): 601–607. And Peterson, Charlotte, PhD, Personal Observations, Bali, Indonesia, 1989.
16. G. Morelli et al., "Cultural variation in infants' sleeping arrangements: Questions of independence," *Developmental Psychology* 28 (1992): 604–613.
17. Richard Ferber, *Solve Your Child's Sleep Problems* (New York City, NY: Fireside, 2006).
18. Paul M. Fleiss, MD, *Sweet Dreams: A Pediatrician's Secrets for Your Child's Good Night's Sleep* (Los Angeles, CA: Lowell House, 2000).

19. Lylah M. Alphonse, "Is Crying it Out Dangerous for Kids?" *Yahoo! Shine /Parenting*, December 16, 2011, http://news.yahoo.com/ is-crying-it-out-dangerous-for-kids.html;ylt=A0SO82Ki_tBVl1A AyX7rFAx.;ylu=X3oDMTByb2lvbXVuBGNvbG8DZ3ExBHBvcw-MxBHZ0aWQDBHNlYwNzcg—.

20. Darcia Narvaez, PhD, "Dangers of 'Crying It Out,'" *Psychology Today: Moral Landscape*, December 11, 2011.

21. Thomas Phelan, "Do You Know Your Parenting Style?" *Brainy Child: All About Child Brain Development*, April 1, 2011. http://www. brainy-child.com.

22. Gordon Neufeld, PhD and Gabor Maté, MD, *Hold On to Your Kids: Why Parents need to Matter More Than Peers* (New York City, NY: Ballantine Books: The Random House Publishing Group, 2006).

23. Nancy Eisenberg, *The Caring Child* (Cambridge, MA: Harvard University Press, 1999).

24. Allport, *A Natural History of Parenting*, 178–179.

25. Neufeld and Maté, *Hold On to Your Kids*.

26. Attachment Parenting International, Mission Statement: "*The Truth is*," last modified August 14, 2015. http://www.attachmentparenting. org/.

27. William Sears, MD and Martha Sears, RN, *The Attachment Parenting Book: A Commonsense Guide to Understanding and Nurturing Your Child* (New York City, NY: Hachette Book Group, 2001).

28. Pam Leo, *Connection Parenting: Parenting Through Connection Instead of Coercion, Through Love Instead of Fear* (Deadwood, Oregon: Wyatt-MacKenzie Publishing, 2005).

29. Leo, *Connection Parenting*, 27.

30. Neufeld and Maté, *Hold On to Your Kids*, 6.

31. Leo, *Connection Parenting*, 29.

32. Stephen H. Bahr, and John P Hoffman, "Parenting Style, Religiosity, Peers, and Adolescent Heavy Drinking," *Journal of Studies on Alcohol and Drugs* Volume 71, Issue 4 (July 2010).

33. Balter, *Parenthood in America*.

34. Noah Webster, *Webster's New Universal Unabridged Dictionary* (New York City, NY: Simon and Schuster, 1983).

35. Webster, *Webster's New Universal Unabridged Dictionary.*
36. Jan Hunt, "The Natural Child Project: Corporal Punishment—10 Reasons Not to Hit Your Kids," American Society for the Positive Care of Children, 2014. http://americanspcc.org/10-reasons-hit-kids/.
37. Robin Grille, *Parenting For A Peaceful World* (New South Wales, Australia: Longueville Media, 2005).
38. Adrienne A. Haeuser, "Swedish Parents Don't Spank," 1989. http://www.neverhitachild.org/haeuser.html.
39. Global Initiative to End All Corporal Punishment of Children, "Ending Legalized violence against children," last modified July 24, 2015. www.endcorporalpunishment.org.
40. Global Initiative: "Ending Legalized violence against children."
41. Wikipedia, "School Corporal Punishment," last modified on August 13, 2015, https://en.wikipedia.org/wiki/School_corporal_punishment.
42. Hillary Rodham Clinton, *It Takes A Village: And Other Lessons Children Teach Us* (New York City, NY: Simon and Schuster, 1996.

## Chapter 5

1. Charlotte Peterson, PhD, "Second That Emotion!" *Child*, June/July 1995.
2. William H. Frey and Muriel Langseth, *Crying: The Mystery of Tears* (Minneapolis, MN: Winston Press, 1985).
3. Peterson, "Second That Emotion!"
4. Rosemary Black, "The Many Faces of Time-Out," *Child*, November 1996.
5. Nancy Shute, "For Kids, Self-Control Factors Into Future Success," National Public Radio, February 14, 2011. http://npr.org/2011/02/14/133629477/for-kids-self-control-factors-into-success.

## Chapter 6

1. Meredith F. Small, *Kids: How Biology and Culture Shape the Way We Raise Young Children* (New York City, NY: Anchor Books, 2001).

2. Doc Childre and Howard Martin, *The Heartmath Solution* (New York City, NY: HarperCollins, 2000).
3. T. R. Verny, MD and Pamela Weintraub, *Pre-Parenting: Nurturing Your Child from Conception* (New York City, NY: Simon & Schuster, 2002).
4. B. Devlin et al., "The Heritability of IQ," *Nature*, 1997, 468–471.
5. BBC News, "Mum's stress is passed to baby in the womb," reported by Michelle Roberts, July 19, 2011. http://www.bbc.co.uk/news/health-14187905.
6. Bruce H. Lipton, PhD, *The Biology of Belief: Unleashing the Power of Consciousness, Matter & Miracles* (Santa Rosa, CA: Mountain of Love/Elite Books, 2005),174.
7. Stanley I. Greenspan, MD and Beryl Lieff Benderly, *The Growth of the Mind: And the Endangered Origins of Intelligence* (New York City, NY: Perseus Books, 1998).
8. Allan Schore, PhD, *Affect Regulation and the Origin of the Self* (Hillsdale, NJ: Lawrence Erlbaum Associates, Inc., 1994).
9. Sue Gerhardt, *Why Love Matters: How affection shapes a baby's brain* (New York City, NY: Brunner-Routledge, 2004), 36.
10. Alex Korb, PhD, "Lick Your Kids: What rats can teach us about parenting," *Psychology Today*. (Post published in PreFrontal Nudity, February 29, 2012). https://www.psychologytoday.com/blog/prefrontal-nudity/201202/lick-your-kids
11. James W. Prescott, PhD, "Affectional bonding for the prevention of violent behaviors: Neurobiological, Psychological and Religious/Spiritual Determinants," in *Violent Behavior, Vol. 1: Assessment & Intervention*, ed. L.J. Hertzberg, et.al., (New York: PMA Publishing Corp. 1990), 110–142.
12. C. Holden, "Child Development: Small Refugees Suffer the Effects of Early Neglect," *Science* 274, no. 5290 (1996): 1076–1077.
13. Maia Szalavitz and Bruce D. Perry, MD, PhD, *Born For Love: Why Empathy is Essential—and Endangered* (New York City, NY: HarperCollins, 2010).
14. Lhamu, personal interview.

15. Daniel Siegel, MD and Tina Payne Bryson, PhD, *The Whole-Brain Child: 12 Revolutionary Strategies to Nurture Your Child's Developing Brain* (New York City, NY: Delacorte Press, 2011).
16. A. Dettling, M. Gunnar, and B. Donzella, "Cortisol Levels of Young Children in full-day childcare centres," *Psychoneuroendrocrinology* 24 (1999): 519–36.
17. A. Dettling et. al., "Quality of care and temperament determine changes in cortisol concentrations over the day for young children in childcare," *Psychoneuroendrocrinology* 25 (2000): 819–36.
18. B. Klimes-Dugan and Megan Gunnar, "Social Regulation of the Adrenocortical Response to Stress in Infants, Children, and Adolescents: Implications for Psychopathology and Education," in *Human Behavior, Learning, and the Developing Brain: Atypical Development,* ed. D. Coch, G. Dawson, and K. Fisher (New York City, NY: Guilford Press, 2007).
19. Neufeld and Maté, MD, *Hold On to Your Kids.*
20. Linda Lantieri and Daniel Goleman, *Building Emotional Intelligence: Practices to Cultivate Inner Resilience in Children* (Electronic University; 1 edition, 2014).
21. Harold Chugani, MD, et al., "Local brain functional activity following early deprivation: a study of post-institutionalized Romanian orphans," *Neuroimage* 14 (2001):1290–1301.
22. William Christeson, Martha Brooks, and Soren Messner-Zidell, "Breaking the Cycle of Child Abuse and Reducing Crime in Oregon," A report for Fight Crime: Invest in Kids Oregon, 2009.
23. Robin Karr-Morse with Meredith S. Wiley, *Scared Sick: The Role of Childhood Trauma in Adult Disease* (Philadelphia, PA: Basic Books, Perseus Books Group, 2012).
24. Karr-Morse, *Scared Sick.*
25. S.R. Dube et al., "Childhood Abuse, Neglect, and Household Dysfunction and the Risk of Illicit Drug Use: The Adverse Childhood Experiences Study," *Pediatrics* 111, no. 3 (March 2003): 564–572.
26. Karr-Morse, *Scared Sick.*
27. Nancy Shute, "Kids Involved in Bullying Grow Up To Be Poorer, Sicker Adults," National Public Radio, August 19, 2013. http://npr.

org/blogs/health/2013/08/19 /213502228/kids-involved-in-bullying-grow-up-to-be-poorer-sicker-adults.

## Chapter 7

1. Madeleine M. Kunin, *The New Feminist Agenda: Defining the Next Revolution for Women, Work, and Family,* (White River Junction, VT: Chelsea Green Publishing, 2012).
2. L.C. Hibel, E. Mercado and J.M. Trumbell, "Parenting stressors and morning cortisol in a sample of working mothers," *Journal of Family Psychology* 26, no. 5 (2012): 738–46. http://www.ncbi.nlm.nih.gov/pubmed/22866929.
3. New York Times, "Paid Maternal Leave: Almost Everywhere, "February 17, 2013. Source: Jody Heymann with Kristen McNeill. *Children's Chances: How Countries Can Move From Surviving to Thriving* (Cambridge, MA: Harvard University Press, 2013). http://www.nytimes.com/imagepages/2013/02/17/opinion/17coontz2-map.html.
4. Kunin, *The New Feminist Agenda.*
5. Tala Al-Hejailan, "Saudi Labor Law and the Rights of Women Employees," *Arab News,* January 24, 2010.
6. United Nations Statistics Division, Table 5g: "Maternity Leave Benefits," updated June 2011. http://unstats.un.org/unsd/default.htm.
7. Anne Lise Ellingsaeter and Arnlaug Leira, eds. *Politicizing Parenthood in Scandinavia: Gender Relations in Welfare States* (Bristol, UK: The Policy Press, 2006).
8. Gillian Witherspoon, Laura Gillen, and Megan Richardson, "Finland: Family Leave Policies" (New Orleans, LA: Tulane University, May 5, 2009). http://www.tulane.edu /~rouxbee/soci626/finland/familyleave.html.
9. Kunin, *The New Feminist Agenda.*
10. Francesca Levy, "Table: The World's Happiest Countries," *Forbes,* July 14, 2010. http://www.forbes.com/2010/07/14/world-happiest-countries-lifestyle-realestate-gallup-table.html.
11. Kunin, *The New Feminist Agenda.*

12. *Connexion* (France's English-Language Newspaper), "Parental leave rules explained," December 2010.
13. Kunin, *The New Feminist Agenda*.
14. Katrin Benhold, "Working (Part-Time) in the 21st Century," *New York Times*, December 30, 2010.
15. Elterngeld und Elternzeit. German Federal Office for Immigrants and Refugees. Retrieved June 25, 2014.
16. Kunin, *The New Feminist Agenda*.
17. Kunin, *The New Feminist Agenda*.
18. Kunin, *The New Feminist Agenda*.
19. Kunin, *The New Feminist Agenda*.
20. Service Canada, "Employment Insurance Maternity and Paternal Benefits," Archived and retrieved from the original on August 22, 2012.
21. Kunin, *The New Feminist Agenda*.
22. Kunin, *The New Feminist Agenda*.
23. Wikipedia "Parental Leave." last modified on 12 July 2015. https://en.wikipedia.org/wiki/Parental_leave.
24. Kunin, *The New Feminist Agenda*.
25. Mark Weinberger, Presentation at White House Summit on Working Families, Washington, DC, June 23, 2014.
26. White House Summit on Working Families, Washington, DC, June 23, 2014. www.workingfamiliessummit.org.
27. White House Summit on Working Families, 2014.
28. Kunin, *The New Feminist Agenda*.
29. White House Summit on Working Families, 2014.
30. State of California Department of Fair Employment and Housing, *Pregnancy Leave*, 2007. www.dfeh.ca.gov/res/docs/Publications/DFEH-186.pdf.
31. Kunin, *The New Feminist Agenda*.
32. Callander, Meryn G. *Why Dads Leave: Insights & Resources for When Partners Become Parents* (Ashville, NC: Akasha Publications, 2012).
33. Steve Biddulph, "A Creche Can't Love Them," *The Herald Sun*, April 7, 1994.
34. Karr-Morse, *Scared Sick*.

35. Moynihan, Carolyn, "Is day care good for babies?" Interview with Ann Manne, *MercatorNet*. August 18, 2006.
36. Anne Manne, *Motherhood*. (Sydney, Australia: Allen and Unwin, 2005).
37. Karr-Morse, *Scared Sick*.
38. Penelope Leach, *Children First* (London, England: Michael Joseph Pub., 1994).
39. Charlotte Peterson, PhD, personal interview with Amy Ripley and Susan Schneider, University of Oregon's Vivian Olum Child Development Center, October 17, 2014.
40. Thomas E. Perez, US Secretary of Labor speaking at the White House Summit on Working Families, Washington DC: June 23, 2014.

## Chapter 8

1. Kim Parker,"5 facts about today's fathers," Pew Research Center: Fact Tank, June 18, 2015. http://www.pewresearch.org/fact-tank/2015/06/18/5-facts-about-todays-fathers/.
2. Anxiety and Depression Association of America, "Understanding the Facts of Anxiety Disorders and Depression is the first step," 2010–2015. http://www.adaa.org/about-adaa/press-room/facts-statistics.
3. White House Summit on Working Families, 2014.
4. ABC News Special, "Barbara Walters: Her Story," July 5, 2014.
5. Barbara Graham, "'Grandma' Gets a Reboot: How boomer women are redefining the role," *AARP Bulletin*, Cover article: September 2014.
6. Graham, "'Grandma' Gets a Reboot".
7. Graham, "'Grandma' Gets a Reboot".
8. Becky Brittain Hicks, PhD and Eric von Schrader, Planet Grandparent Workshop: "Teaching Grandparents to Help Parents and Babies Thrive," 2011. www.planetgrandparent.com.
9. Sally Abrams, "Three Generations Under One Roof," *AARP Bulletin*, April 2013, 53(3): 16–20.

# Appendix

1. Barbara Findeisen, presidential address at Association for Pre & Perinatal Psychology and Health: 11th International Congress, "Birth, Brain, and Bonding: The Psychology and Science of Attachment," San Francisco, CA, December 4, 2003.
2. *Reducing Infant Mortality*, directed by Debby Takikawa.
3. *Reducing Infant Mortality*, directed by Debby Takikawa.
4. Findeisen, presidential address
5. Findeisen, presidential address
6. Alliance for Transforming the Lives of Children, "Bonding and Attachment in the Family," North American Invitational Summit, Santa Barbara, CA: March 27-30, 2003.
7. ABC News, news broadcast, September 19, 2000.
8. ABC News, news broadcast, September 19, 2000.
9. U.S. Surgeon General, "Children and Mental Health," in *Mental Health: A Report of the Surgeon General*, Chapter 3 (Rockville, MD: National Institute of Mental Health, 1999).
10. National Mental Health Association, "Mental Health Disorders Are Common: Treatment is Not," Mental Health America, 2003. http://www.nmha.org/.
11. *Bully*, directed by Katy Butler (New York City, NY: The Bully Project, 2012). DVD. Movie trailer: www.thebullyproject.com.
12. Neufeld and Maté, MD, *Hold On to Your Kids*.
13. National Mental Health Association, "Mental Health Disorders Are Common
14. ABC News, News Broadcast, September 19, 2000.
15. National Center for Children Exposed to Violence, Yale University Child Study Center, New Haven, CT. November 29, 2003. http://medicine.yale.edu/childstudycenter /cvtc/.
16. National Center for Children Exposed to Violence.
17. National Center for Children Exposed to Violence.
18. William Damon, *Greater Expectations: Overcoming the Culture of Indulgence in our Homes and Schools* (New York City, NY: Free Press Paperbacks, 1995).

19. Christeson, Brooks, and Messner-Zidell, "Breaking the Cycle of Child Abuse and Reducing Crime in Oregon." A report for Fight Crime: Invest in Kids Oregon, 2009.

# Bibliography

ABC News. News Broadcast. September 19, 2000.

ABC News Special. "Barbara Walters: Her Story." July 5, 2014.

Abrams, Sally. "Three Generations Under One Roof," *AARP Bulletin,* April 2013, 53(3): 16–20.

Agency for Healthcare Research and Quality, "Breastfeeding and Maternal and Infant Health Outcomes in Developed Countries," Evidence Report, April 2007, http//www.ahrq.gov/clinic.epcarch.htm.

Al-Hejailan, Tala,."Saudi Labor Law and the Rights of Women Employees," *Arab News,* January 24, 2010.

Alliance for Transforming the Lives of Children. "Bonding and Attachment in the Family." North American Invitational Summit, Santa Barbara, CA: March 27-30, 2003.

Allport, Susan. *A Natural History of Parenting: A Naturalist Looks at Parenting In the Animal World and Ours.* Bloomington, IN: iUniverse, 2003.

Allport, Susan. *A Natural History of Parenting: From Emperor Penguins to Reluctant Ewes, a Naturalist Looks at Parenting in the Animal World and Ours.* New York City, NY: Harmony Books, 1997.

Alphonse, Lylah M. "Is Crying it Out Dangerous for Kids?" *Yahoo! Shine/Parenting,* December 16, 2011. http://news.yahoo.com/is-crying-it-out-dangerous-for-kids. Html; ylt=A0SO82Ki_tBVl1AAyX-7rFAx.;ylu=X3oDMTByb2lvbXVuBGNvbG8DZ3ExBHBvcwMx-BHZ0aWQDBHNlYwNzcg--.

American Academy of Pediatrics. Policy Statement: "Breastfeeding and the Use of Human Milk," *Pediatrics* 115 no. 2 (February 2005): 496–506.

American Academy of Pediatrics. Resolution #67SC, "Divesting From Formula Marketing in Pediatric Care," Breastfeeding Initiatives, November 25, 2011. https://www2.aap.org /breastfeeding/files/pdf/DivestingfromFormulaMarketinginPediatricCare.pdf

Aney, Matthew, MD. "Babywise advice linked to dehydration, failure to thrive." 1995. http://www.ezzo.info/resources/timeline/81-timeline/107-babywise-advice-linked-to-dehydration-failure-to-thrive.

Anxiety and Depression Association of America. "Understanding the Facts of Anxiety Disorders and Depression is the first step." 2010-2015. http://www.adaa.org/about-adaa /press-room/facts-statistics.

Association for Prenatal and Perinatal Psychology and Health. "Welcome Your Baby In With 60 Minutes, Skin-to-Skin," Advocate Reference Card, 2010. http://www.birthpsychology.com.

Attachment Parenting International, Mission Statement: "*The Truth is*," Last modified August 14, 2015. http://www.attachmentparenting.org/.

Australian Association of Infant Mental Health. Position Paper 1: "Controlled Crying." March 2004. http://www.aaimhi.org/inewsfiles/controlled_crying.pdf.

Baby Friendly USA. "Implementing the UNICEF/WHO Baby Friendly Hospital Initiative in the U.S." Last modified 2012. http://www.baby-friendlyusa.

Bahr, Stephen H. and John P. Hoffman. "Parenting Style, Religiosity, Peers, and Adolescent Heavy Drinking," *Journal of Studies on Alcohol and Drugs*, Volume 71, Issue 4 (July 2010).

Balter, Lawrence. *Parenthood in America: An Encyclopedia, Volume 1*, Santa Barbara, CA: ABC-CLIO, Inc.,2000.

BBC News. "Mum's stress is passed to baby in the womb," Reported by Michelle Roberts, July 19, 2011. http://www.bbc.co.uk/news/health-14187905.

Bell, Silvia M., and Mary D. Salter Ainsworth, "Infant crying and maternal responsiveness," *Child Development* 43 (1972): 1171–90.

Benhold, Katrin. "Working (Part-Time) in the 21st Century." *New York Times:* December 30, 2010.

Biddulph, Steve."A Creche Can't Love Them," *The Herald Sun,*. April 7, 1994.

Black, Rosemary. "The Many Faces of Time-Out." *Child*, Volume 11, No. 9, November 1996.

Blaffer Hrdy, Sarah. *Mother Nature: Maternal Instincts and How They Shape the Human Species*. New York City, NY: Ballantine Publishing Group, 2000.

Bretherton, Inge. "The Origins of Attachment Theory: John Bowlby and Mary Ainsworth," *Developmental Psychology 28*, (1992): 759–775.

Brown, Brené, PhD. *The Gifts of Imperfection: Let Go of Who You Think You're Supposed to Be and Embrace Who You Are.* Center City, MN: Hazelden, 2010.

Buckley, Sarah J., MD. *Gentle Birth, Gentle Mothering: The Wisdom and Science of Gentle Choices in Pregnancy, Birth, and Parenting.* Australia: One Moon Press, 2005.

*Bully.* Directed by Katy Butler. New York City, NY: The Bully Project, 2012. DVD. Movie trailer: www.thebullyproject.com.

Callander, Meryn G. *Why Dads Leave: Insights & Resources for When Partners Become Parents.* Ashville, NC: Akasha Publications, 2012.

Carpenter, Russ and Blyth Carpenter. *The Blessings of Bhutan.* Honolulu, HI: University of Hawai'i Press, 2002.

Childre, Doc, and Howard Martin. *The Heartmath Solution.* New York City, NY: HarperCollins, 2000.

Choegyal, Rinchen Khando. Personal Interview. Dharamsala, India, December 1994.

Christeson, William, Martha Brooks, and Soren Messner-Zidell. "Breaking the Cycle of Child Abuse and Reducing Crime in Oregon." A report for Fight Crime: Invest in Kids Oregon, 2009.

Chugani, Harold, MD, M. Behen, O. Muzik, C. Juhasz, F. Nagy, and D. Chugani. "Local brain functional activity following early deprivation: a study of post-institutionalized Romanian orphans." *Neuroimage* 14 (2001): 1290-1301.

Clark, Mary E. *In Search of Human Nature.* New York City, NY: Routledge, 2002.

Clark, Mary E. Personal Conversation. Eugene, OR, 2011.

Clinton, Hillary Rodham. *It Takes A Village: And Other Lessons Children Teach Us.* New York City, NY: Simon and Schuster,1996.

*Connexion* (France's English-Language Newspaper). "Parental leave rules explained," December 2010.

Crawford, M. "Parenting Practices in the Basque Country: Implications of Infant and Childhood Sleeping Location for Personality Development." *Ethos* 22, no. 1 (1994): 42–82.

Damon, William. *Greater Expectations: Overcoming the Culture of Indulgence in our Homes and Schools.* New York City, NY: Free Press Paperbacks,1995.

Davis, Wendy, PhD. "Perinatal Mood Disorders." Presentation, Lane County, Oregon: May 8, 2006. http://www.babybluesconnection.org.

*Delivery Self-Attachment.* Directed by Lennart Righard. Los Angeles, CA: Geddes Productions. 1995. Video.

Dentan, Robert Knox. *The Semai: A Nonviolent People of Malaya.* New York: Holt, Rinehart and Winston,1968.

Dettling, A., M. Gunnar, and B. Donzella. "Cortisol Levels of Young Children in full-day childcare centres." *Psychoneuroendrocrinology* 24 (1999): 519–36.

Dettling, A., S. Parker, S. Lane, A. Sebanc and M. Gunnar. "Quality of care and temperament determine changes in cortisol concentrations over the day for young children in childcare." *Psychoneuroendrocrinology* 25 (2000): 819–36.

Devlin, B., M. Daniels, et.al. "The Heritability of IQ." *Nature 388* (1997): 468–471.

Dube, S. R., V. Felitti, M. Dong, D. Chapman, W. Giles, and R. Anda. "Childhood Abuse, Neglect, and Household Dysfunction and the Risk of Illicit Drug Use: The Adverse Childhood Experiences Study." *Pediatrics* 111, no. 3 (March 2003): 564–572.

Eisenberg,Nancy. *The Caring Child.* Cambridge, MA: Harvard University Press,1999.

Eisler, Riane. *The Chalice and the Blade.* New York City. NY: HarperCollins, 1988.

Ellingsaeter, Anne Lise and Arnlaug Leira, eds. *Politicizing Parenthood in Scandinavia: Gender Relations in Welfare States.* Bristol, UK: The Policy Press, 2006.

Elterngeld und Elternzeit. German Federal Office for Immigrants and Refugees. Retrieved June 25, 2014.

Erikson, Erik. *Childhood and Society.* New York City: NY: WW Norton & Company, 1950.

Ezzo, Gary. *On Becoming Babywise.* Sisters, Oregon: Multnomah Publishers, 1998.

Ezzo, Gary and Robert Bucknam. *On Becoming Babywise: Giving Your Infant the Gift of Nighttime Sleep.* Sisters, Oregon: Multnomah Publishers, 2006.

Ferber, Richard. *Solve Your Child's Sleep Problems.* New York City, NY: Fireside, 2006.

Ferrucci, Piero. *The Power of Kindness: The Unexpected Benefits of Leading a Compassionate Life.* London, England: Penguin Books, 2006.

Findeisen, Barbara. Presidential Address at Association for Pre & Perinatal Psychology and Health: 11th International Congress. "Birth, Brain, and Bonding: The Psychology and Science of Attachment." San Francisco, CA, December 4, 2003.

Fleiss, Paul M., MD. *Sweet Dreams: A Pediatrician's Secrets for Your Child's Good Night's Sleep.* Los Angeles, CA: Lowell House, 2000.

Follmi, Olivier, and Danielle Follmi. *Offerings: Spiritual Wisdom to Change Your Life.* New York City, NY: Stewart, Tabori & Chang, 2002.

Formon, Samuel J. "Infant Feeding in the 20th Century: Formula and Beikost." *Journal of Nutrition* 131 (2001): 4095–4205.

Frey, William H. and Muriel Langseth. *Crying: The Mystery of Tears.* Minneapolis, MN: Winston Press, 1985.

Gandri, Nyoman. Personal Interview. Payogan, Bali, Indonesia, 2002.

Gartner, L.M. et. al. Policy Statement: "Breastfeeding and the use of human milk." *Pediatrics* 115, no.2 (2005): 496–506.

Gerhardt, Sue. *Why Love Matters: How affection shapes a baby's brain.* New York City, NY: Brunner-Routledge, 2004.

Global Initiative to End All Corporal Punishment of Children. "Ending Legalized violence against children." Last modified July 24, 2015. www. endcorporalpunishment.org.

Graham, Barbara. "'Grandma' Gets a Reboot: How boomer women are redefining the role." *AARP Bulletin,* Cover article: September 2014.

Greenspan, Stanley I., MD and Beryl Lieff Benderly. *The Growth of the Mind: And the Endangered Origins of Intelligence.* New York City, NY: Perseus Books, 1998.

Grille, Robin. *Parenting For A Peaceful World.* New South Wales, Australia: Longueville Media, 2005.

Guttmacher Institute. "Facts on Unintended Pregnancy in the United States." January 2012. www.guttmacher.org/pubs/FB-Unintended-Pregnancy-US.html.

Haeuser, Adrienne A. "Swedish Parents Don't Spank." 1989. http://www.neverhitachild.org/haeuser.html.

Harris, Lynn. "Spare the quarter-inch plumbing supply line, spoil the child." May 25, 2006. http://www.salon.com/life/feature/2006/05/25/the_pearls.

Healthy Babies, Healthy Communities. "Safe Sleep." Flyer by a grant from the CJ Foundation for SIDS. Lane County, Oregon, 2009. www.lane-county.org/prevention.

Heinowitz, Jack. *Fathering Right from the Start: Straight Talk about Pregnancy, Birth and Beyond.* Novato, CA: New World Library, 2001.

Hibel, L. C., Mercado, E., Trumbell, J. M. "Parenting stressors and morning cortisol in a sample of working mothers." *Journal of Family Psychology* 26, no. 5 (2012): 738–46. http://www.ncbi.nlm.nih.gov/pubmed/22866929.

Hicks, Becky Brittain, PhD and Eric von Schrader. Planet Grandparent Workshop: "Teaching Grandparents to Help Parents and Babies Thrive," 2011. www.planetgrandparent.com.

Holden, C. "Child Development: Small Refugees Suffer the Effects of Early Neglect." *Science* 274, no. 5290 (1996): 1076-1077.

Holt, Emmett L., MD. *The Care and Feeding of Children: A Catechism for the Use of Mothers and Children's Nurses.* Public domain in the USA, (1907).

Houser, Patrick M. "Breast is Best . . . for Dads too!" La Leche League Magazine: *New Beginnings*, August 2009.

Houser, Patrick M. "The Science of Father Love." Association for Prenatal and Perinatal Psychology and Health, 2011. https://birthpsychology.com/free-article/science-father-love.

Hunt, Jan. "The Natural Child Project: Corporal Punishment—10 Reasons Not to Hit Your Kids." American Society for the Positive Care of Children. 2014. http://americanspcc.org/10-reasons-hit-kids/.

Infant Massage USA. "Benefits of Infant Massage." 2011. www.infantmassageusa/learn-to-massage-your-baby/benefits-of-infant-massage/.

International Childbirth Education Association. *Cesarean Fact Sheet.* 1995–1998. http://www.childbirth.org/section/CSFact.html.

Johnson, Nathanael. "As early elective births increase so do health risks for mother, child." California Watch: December 26, 2010. http://californiawatch.org.

Karen, Robert. *Becoming Attached: First Relationships and How They Shape Our Capacity to Love.* New York City, NY: Oxford University Press, 1994.

Karr-Morse, Robin with Meredith S. Wiley. *Scared Sick: The Role of Childhood Trauma in Adult Disease.* Philadelphia, PA: Basic Books, Perseus Books Group, 2012.

Karta, Ketut. Personal Interview. Penestanan, Bali, Indonesia, August 2002.

Kato, Norihiro. "Japan's Break with Peace," *The New York Times.* July 16, 2014.

Kikuchi, Naho. Personal Interview. Tokyo, Japan, September 2002.

Klaus, Marshall H., MD and John H. Kennel. *Maternal-infant Bonding.* St. Louis, MO: C. V. Mosby Co., 1976.

Klaus, Marshall H., MD and Phyllis H. Klaus. *Your Amazing Newborn.* New York City, NY: HarperCollins Publishers, 1998.

Klimes-Dugan, B and Megan Gunnar. "Social Regulation of the Adrenocortical Response to Stress in Infants, Children, and Adolescents: Implications for Psychopathology and Education." In *Human Behavior, Learning, and the Developing Brain: Atypical Development,* edited by D. Coch, G. Dawson, and K. Fisher. New York City, NY: Guilford Press, 2007.

Korb, Alex, PhD. "Lick Your Kids: What rats can teach us about parenting." *Psychology Today.* (Post published in PreFrontal Nudity, February 29, 2012). https://www.psychologytoday.com/blog/prefrontal-nudity/201202/lick-your-kids

*Kundun.* Directed by Martin Scorsese. Burbank, CA: Touchstone Pictures. 1997. DVD.

Kunin, Madeleine M. *The New Feminist Agenda: Defining the Next Revolution for Women, Work, and Family.* White River Junction, VT: Chelsea Green Publishing, 2012.

Lantieri, Linda, and Daniel Goleman. *Building Emotional Intelligence: Practices to Cultivate Inner Resilience in Children.* Electronic University; 1 edition, 2014.

Leach, Penelope. *Children First.* London, England: Michael Joseph Pub., 1994.

Lee, K. "The Crying Patterns of Korean Infants & Related Factors." *Developmental Medicine & Child Neurology* 36 (1994): 601–607.

Leo, Pam. *Connection Parenting: Parenting Through Connection Instead of Coercion, Through Love Instead of Fear.* Deadwood, Oregon: Wyatt-MacKenzie Publishing, 2005.

Levy, Francesca. "Table: The World's Happiest Countries." *Forbes,* July 14, 2010. http://www.forbes.com/2010/07/14/world-happiest-countries-lifestyle-realestate-gallup-table.html.

Lhamu, Mimi, MD. Personal Interview. Thimphu, Bhutan, February 25, 2004.

Lim, Robin. Personal Interview. Banjar Nyuh Kuning, Bali, March 31, 2004.

Lipton, Bruce H., PhD. *The Biology of Belief: Unleashing the Power of Consciousness, Matter & Miracles.* Santa Rosa, CA: Mountain of Love/Elite Books, 2005.

Littman, H., S. VanderBrug Medendorp, and J. Goldfarb. "The Decision to Breastfeed: The Importance of Fathers' Approval." *Clinical Pediatrics, 33, no.*4 (1994): 214–219.

MacEnulty, Pat. "Oh Baby: Ina May Gaskin on the Medicalization of Birth." *The Sun,* January 2012, 5–13.

Maiden, Ann Hubbell, and Edie Farwell. *The Tibetan Art of Parenting: From Before Conception Through Early Childhood.* Somerville, MA: Wisdom Publications, 1997.

Manne, Anne. *Motherhood.* Sydney, Australia: Allen and Unwin, 2005.

McKenna, James J., Sarah Mosko, Claiborne Dungy, and Jan McAninch. "Sleep and Arousal Patterns of Co-Sleeping Human Mother-Infant Pairs: A Preliminary Physiological Study with Implications for the Study of the Sudden Infant Death Syndrome (SIDS)." *American Journal of Physical Anthropology,* 82 no.3 (1990): 331–347.

McKenna, James J., PhD. *Sleeping with Your Baby: A Parent's Guide to Cosleeping.* Washington, DC: Platypus Media; 1 edition, 2007.

Bibliography

McKenna, James J., PhD. and Lee T. Gettler. "Mother-Infant Cosleeping with Breastfeeding in the Western Industrialized Context: A Bicultural Perspective." In *Textbook of Human Lactation,* edited by T. W. Hale and P. E. Hartmann. Amarillo, TX: Hale Publishing, 2007.

Mendoza, S. P., and W. A Mason. "Attachment Relationships in New World Primates." In *The Integrative Neurobiology of Affiliation,* edited by C. S. Carter, I. I. Lederhendler, and B. Kirkpatrick, 93-100. Cambridge, MA: MIT Press, 1999.

Morelli, G., Rogoff, B., Oppenheim, D., and Goldsmith, D. "Cultural variation in infants' sleeping arrangements: Questions of independence." *Developmental Psychology* 28 (1992): 604–613.

Moynihan, Carolyn. "Is day care good for babies?" Interview with Ann Manne. *MercatorNet.* August 18, 2006.

Narok, Made. Personal Interview. Penestanan, Bali, Indonesia, July 2002.

Narvaez, Darcia, PhD. "Dangers of 'Crying It Out.'" *Psychology Today: Moral Landscape,* December 11, 2011.

National Center for Children Exposed to Violence. Yale University Child Study Center, New Haven, CT. November 29, 2003. http://medicine. yale.edu/childstudycenter/cvtc/.

National Institute of Child Health and Human Development. "High C-section rate may have something to do with impatience." *Los Angeles Times,* August 30, 2010.

National Institute of Child Health and Human Development. Public Education Campaign: "Safe to Sleep." Last modified January 2, 2015. http://www.nichd.nih.gov /sts/Pages/default.aspx.

National Mental Health Association. "Mental Health Disorders Are Common: Treatment is Not." Mental Health America, 2003. http://www. nmha.org/.

Nelson, Desiree, RN, IBCLC. Written Personal Communication. December 12, 2011.

Neufeld, Gordon, PhD and Gabor Maté, MD. *Hold On to Your Kids: Why Parents need to Matter More Than Peers.* New York City, NY: Ballantine Books: The Random House Publishing Group, 2006.

New York Times, "Paid Maternal Leave: Almost Everywhere," February 17, 2013. Source: Jody Heymann with Kristen McNeill. *Children's*

*Chances: How Countries Can Move From Surviving to Thriving.* Cambridge, MA: Harvard University Press, 2013. http://www.nytimes.com/imagepages/2013/02/17/opinion/17coontz2-map.html.

Newman, Jack, MD. "The Importance of Skin to Skin Contact." International Breastfeeding Center. 2009. http://www.nbci.ca/index.php?option=comcontent&id=82:the-importance-of-skin-to-skin-contact-&Itemid=17

Page, Eric. "Benjamin Spock, World's Pediatrician, Dies at 94," New York Times, Network, March 17, 1998. http://learning.blogs.nytimes.com/.

Parker, Kim. "5 facts about today's fathers." Pew Research Center: Fact Tank. June 18, 2015. http://www.pewresearch.org/fact-tank/2015/06/18/5-facts-about-todays-fathers/.

Pearce, Joseph Chilton, and Bruce H. Lipton. "The Evolution of Biology and Development of Spiritual Intelligence." Post Congress Workshop: Association for Prenatal and Perinatal Psychology and Health (APPPAH) 10th International Congress. San Francisco, CA, 2001.

Pearls, Michael, and Debi Pearls. *To Train Up A Child.* Pleasantville, TN: No Greater Joy Ministries, 1994.

Perez, Thomas E. US Secretary of Labor speaking at the White House Summit on Working Families, Washington DC: June 23, 2014.

Peterson, Charlotte, PhD. "Second That Emotion!" *Child*, cover article June/July 1995.

Peterson, Charlotte, PhD. Personal Observations. Bali, Indonesia, 1989, 1992, 2000, 2002, and 2004.

Peterson, Charlotte, PhD. Personal Interview with Amy Ripley, Director and Susan Schneider, Supervisor of Young Age Groups at the University of Oregon's Vivian Olum Child Development Center. October 17, 2014.

Phelan, Thomas. "Do You Know Your Parenting Style?" *Brainy Child: All About Child Brain Development.* April 1, 2011. http://www.brainychild.com.

Prescott, James W., PhD. "Affectional bonding for the prevention of violent behaviors: Neurobiological, Psychological and Religious/Spiritual Determinants." In *Violent Behavior, Vol. 1: Assessment & Intervention*, edited by L. J. Hertzberg, et.al., 110–142. New York: PMA Publishing Corp. 1990.

Prescott, James W., PhD. "The Origins of Human Love and Violence." *Journal of Prenatal & Perinatal Psychology & Health* 10, no. 3 (1996): 143–188.

Ratna, Wayan. Personal Interview. Ubud, Bali, Indonesia, August, 2002.

*Reducing Infant Mortality.* Directed by Debby Takikawa. Santa Barbara, CA: Hana Peace Works, 2009. DVD.

Rein, Steve. "Evaluating Ezzo Programs." Last modified 2013. http://www.ezzo.info.

Rhodes, Jeane, PhD. *The Birth of Hope: a unique novel.* Charleston, SC: CreateSpace Independent Publishing Platform, 2009.

Schore, Allan, PhD. *Affect Regulation and the Origin of the Self.* Hillsdale, NJ: Lawrence Erlbaum Associates, Inc., 1994.

Sears, William, MD and Martha Sears, RN. *The Attachment Parenting Book: A Commonsense Guide to Understanding and Nurturing Your Child.* New York City, NY: Hachette Book Group, 2001.

Sears, William, MD, Robert Sears, MD, James Sears, MD, and Martha Sears, RN. *The Baby Sleep Book: The Complete Guide to a Good Night's Rest for the Whole Family.* Boston, MA: Little, Brown and Company, 2005.

Service Canada. "Employment Insurance Maternity and Paternal Benefits." Archived and retrieved from the original on August 22, 2012.

Shute, Nancy. "For Kids, Self-Control Factors Into Future Success." National Public Radio. February 14, 2011. http://npr.org/2011/02/14/133629477/for-kids-self-control-factors-into-success.

Shute, Nancy. "Kids Involved in Bullying Grow Up To Be Poorer, Sicker Adults." National Public Radio. August 19, 2013. http://npr.org/blogs/health/2013/08/19/213502228 /kids-involved-in-bullying-grow-up-to-be-poorer-sicker-adults.

Siegel, Daniel, MD and Mary Hartzell, MEd. *Parenting From The Inside Out.* New York City, NY: Penguin Group (USA) Inc., 2003.

Siegel, Daniel, MD and Tina Payne Bryson, PhD. *The Whole-Brain Child: 12 Revolutionary Strategies to Nurture Your Child's Developing Brain.* New York City, NY: Delacorte Press, 2011.

Small, Meredith F. *Kids: How Biology and Culture Shape the Way We Raise Young Children.* New York City, NY: Anchor Books, 2001.

Somé, Sobonfu E. *Welcoming Spirit Home: Ancient African Teachings to Celebrate Children and Community.* Novato, CA: New World Library, 1999.

Spock, Benjamin. *The Common Sense Book of Baby and Child Care.* New York City, NY: Duell, Sloan, and Pearce, 1946.

State of California Department of Fair Employment and Housing. *Pregnancy Leave.* 2007. www.dfeh.ca.gov/res/docs/Publications/DFEH-186.pdf.

Szalavitz, Maia and Bruce D. Perry, MD, PhD. *Born For Love: Why Empathy is Essential—and Endangered.* New York City, NY: HarperCollins, 2010.

Taylor, S. E., L. C. Klein, B. P. Lewis, T. L. Gruenewald, R. A. R. Gurung, and J. A. Updegraff. "Female Responses to Stress: Tend and Befriend, Not Fight or Flight." *Psychological Review,* 107, no. 3 (2000): 411-429.

*The First Years Last Forever.* Directed by Rob Reiner. Nashville, TN: Parents Action for Children, 2005. DVD.

US Surgeon General. "Children and Mental Health." In *Mental Health: A Report of the Surgeon General,* Chapter 3. Rockville, MD: National Institute of Mental Health, 1999.

United Nations Statistics Division. Table 5g: "Maternity Leave Benefits." Updated June 2011. http://unstats.un.org/unsd/default.htm.

Vennemann, M. M., T. Banjanowski, B. Brinkmann, G. Jorch, K. Yucesan, C. Sauerland, E. A. Mitchell, and the GeSID Study Group. "Does Breast-feeding Reduce the Risk of Sudden Infant Death Syndrome." *Pediatrics, 123* (2009): *e406-e410.*

Verny, T. R. MD, and Pamela Weintraub. *Pre-Parenting: Nurturing Your Child from Conception.* New York City, NY: Simon & Schuster, 2002.

Webster, Noah..*Webster's New Universal Unabridged Dictionary.* New York City, NY: Simon and Schuster, 1983.

Weinberger, Mark. Presentation at White House Summit on Working Families. Washington, DC, June 23, 2014.

White House Summit on Working Families, Washington, DC, June 23, 2014. www.workingfamiliessummit.org.

Widstrom, A. M., W. Wahlburg, A. S. Matthiesen. "Short-term effects of early suckling and touch of the nipple on maternal behavior." *Early Human Development* 21 (1990): 153-163.

Wikipedia. "Gross National Happiness." Last Modified August 10, 2015. http://en.wikipedia.org/wiki/Gross_national_happiness.

Wikipedia "Parental Leave." Last modified on 12 July 2015. https://en.wikipedia.org/wiki/Parental_leave.

Wikipedia. "School Corporal Punishment." Last Modified on August 13, 2015. https://en.wikipedia.org/wiki/School_corporal_punishment.

Witherspoon, Gillian, Laura Gillen, and Megan Richardson. "Finland: Family Leave Policies." New Orleans, LA: Tulane University, May 5, 2009. http://www.tulane.edu /~rouxbee/soci626/finland/familyleave.html.

*Women of Tibet: Gyalyum Chemo The Great Mother.* Directed by Rosemary Rawcliff. San Francisco, CA: Frame of Mind Films, 2006. DVD.

Wootton, Barbara, Mary D. Salter Ainsworth, R. G. Andry, Robert G. Harlow, S. Lebovici, Margaret Mead, Diane G. Prugh "Deprivation of Maternal Care: A Reassessment of Its Effects." Geneva, Switzerland: *World Health Organization, Public Health Papers*, No.14 1962: pp 255-266. http://apps.who.int/iris/handle/10665/37819.

World Health Organization. "Global Strategy for Infant and Young Child Feeding." Geneva, Switzerland: World Health Organization and UNICEF. 2003.

World Health Organization. "Nutrition: Exclusive Breastfeeding." 2011. http://www.who.int /nutrition/topics/exclusive_breast-feeding/en/.

# Acknowledgments

There are so many people, places, and events that made it possible for this information to be shared. I thank them all. Some of those to which I offer my deepest heartfelt gratitude are:

- The people from peaceful cultures who shared their wisdom and personal stories with me: in Bhutan with Mimi Lhamu, MD; in Japan with Nahou Kikuchi; and in Bali with Wayan Ratna, Ketut Karta, Nyoman Gandri, and my "Balinese son," Made Narok, who for twenty-five years has provided me with endless enthusiastic support; and from the Tibetan community, Rinchen Khando Choegyal, minister of education in the Dalai Lama's Tibetan Government in Exile, whose commitment to how much babies need inspired me to write this book.
- Gen Y Parents for sharing their intimate heartwarming stories of lifestyle changes they are making to help meet the early needs of their infants and toddlers along with bringing extended family members back together for caregiving and support. And the Shaver Family for their willingness to disclose the countless difficulties and triumphs in their journey from international adoptions to securely-attached loving relationships with their children.
- Amy Ripley and Susan Schneider who graciously provided information and a walk-though at the University of Oregon Vivian Olum Child Development Center, a state of the art day care program that does it's best to understand and attempt to meet the needs of infants and toddlers.
- Peter Yarrow, singer, songwriter, cofounder of Peter, Paul and Mary, and founder of Operation Respect, an educational and anti-bullying advocacy group; Robin Karr-Morse, author of *Sacred Sick: The Role of Childhood Trauma in Adult Disease* and *Ghosts from the Nursery: Tracing the Roots of Violence*; Michael Trout, director of the Infant-Parent Institute in Illinois; Christof Plothe, DO, Open Mind Academy Bleichstrasse, Germany; Rupert Linder, MD, past president of the

International Society of Pre and Perinatal Psychology and Medicine; Gayle Chisholm, marketing director for KLCC radio in Eugene, Oregon; Rachel Gottgetreu, Portland, Oregon elementary school teacher and new mother; and Mary E. Clark, PhD, author and professor emeritus of Biology and Conflict Resolution at George Mason University for their very generous and thoughtful endorsements of this book.

- My professional editors for their indispensible contributions and insightful observations: Elizabeth Lyons, Evelyn Fazio, Lee Haroun, and my very first, Mary Cummings, who didn't forget my work after moving to NYC. Her enthusiasm years later connected me with Rachel Vogel, my excellent Literary Agent at Waxman Leavell, who believed in this book and helped it become published.

- My loyal Millennial Generation editors, Shane Peterson, MD, Emily Watters, DC (who also provided the beautiful drawings of the brain), and Kendall Smith. A special thanks to Jacob Madden who was always available to help with discussing issues, endless editing, and creating my wonderful website www.growingkindkids.com.

- Julia Abramoff, my editor at Skyhorse Publishing, who understands the value of growing kind kids and has been committed to having this knowledge in print.

- University students from around the world who have lived in my home offering endless support along with help caring for the house and pets: Yusuf Akamoglu, Buket Ertürk, Anna Fay, Carola Frank, Nihal Jambotkar, Corey Johnson, PhD, Yu Lha, and Sussan Voyteshonock.

- Carl Peterson, PhD, who fathered our beautiful children and helped make our amazing travel adventures possible.

- My dear friends and family who encouraged me every step of the way: Abdul Blair, Emily K. Peterson, Kevin Burns, Erik Verdouw, PT, Candy Callan, Bobbie Cirel, Dee Gribben, the Groussman Clan, Dick and Marje Takei, PhD. My loving Soul Sisters: Alice Blankenship, Marian Blankenship, Katy Bloch, Rachel Gottgetreu, Sophie Bloch, and Amber Lippert. My caring neighbor, Michelle Mickelson, for coordinating our daily walks and my pup's romps with Lucy the retriever; they greatly helped Sahalie tolerate all those long hours lying under the computer table. Thanks Sahalie for your patience . . .

- Robert Blair, my devoted corner man who was consistently there throughout the writing of this book to patch me up, give me pep talks, make me laugh, and put me back in the computer chair whenever I lost confidence.

My precious son and daughter, Shane Peterson, MD, and Emily Watters, DC, for their continuous loving support, and for being amazing world travel companions throughout their childhoods, always opening doors and hearts wherever we went. I'm so very proud of their own professional commitments to making the world a healthier, kinder, and gentler place.

My fantastic retreat cabin on Odell Lake, in the Oregon Cascades, which has provided a sanctuary of beauty and continual spiritual renewal during so many long days and nights of writing over the past six years.